SURVIVAL!

Live Off the Land
in the City
and Country

D1528272

SURVIVAL!

Live Off the Land in the City and Country

by Ragnar Benson
with Devon Christensen

Illustrations by David Bjorkman

CITADEL PRESS   SECAUCUS, N. J.

Table of Contents

Introduction

First of all, I want to warn you that this is not just another "eat roots and berries" book. *Live Off the Land in the City and Country* is about long-term survival under emergency and/or relatively primitive conditions. But please do not jump to conclusions, because at this point my definition of *survival* is probably quite different from your own. Also, our definitions of *emergency conditions* might vary considerably. In my opinion, the greatest danger our western societies face today is a complete economic collapse. But any catastrophe, worldwide or localized, may cut off people from normal supply routes and leave them high and dry. Access to survival information can avert total helplessness.

Your definition of *survival* may be muddled by the suggestions of what I call "pure" survival writers. These pious fellows would have us believe that useful survival techniques are inextricably tied in with wilderness conditions; and that wild plants can provide most of the food you will need to stay alive; further, that you need down sleeping bags, nylon packs and tents, fancy freeze-dried food, special aluminum tools, stoves, lanterns, and so on, just to survive.

I say that most of this is nonsense. Before reading any further, you must clear your mind of these preconceptions. Be forewarned that I will not discuss how to survive a once-a-year three-day hike on the Appalachian Trail. But in fact, this is the basic approach presented in other books about living from nature's harvest.

My own survival program is based on: 1) logic; 2) physical laws; and 3) improvisation. Using these three keys, you *can* survive in old-time style and comfort, in apparently hopeless situations.

Here are some examples of how these three keys figure in my survival program:

1

Logic

We often hear economists and financial experts advise survivalists to invest in gold and diamonds as a hedge against currency failure, anarchy, etcetera. Yet logic tells us that your money is better invested in .22 rifles, ammunition, sewing needles, and similar durable goods, if a future collapse is your main concern. Think about it. When the time comes, other survivors will laugh at people who want to barter their precious gold for guns. When a deal like this is over, as Kurt Saxon says, one of the traders will have both gold and gun—and it's not going to be the gold-hoarder.

Physical Laws

I refer primarily to "Benson's Law" of thermodynamics. Basically, this homemade law states that it is unacceptable to put more pure energy into a given project than can be gained from it. In other words, it is foolish to spend all day rooting around for awful-tasting tubers with minimal nutritional properties, when it is 100 times easier and smarter to set up a line of simple box traps and wire snares that will produce wild, wholesome game animals day after day. Very little effort is expended after the trap line is set up. All you need to do thereafter is walk by the traps every day or so, check them, collect any harvested critters, and reset the traps. In case you do not already know this, fresh red meat has more inherent protein and vitamin value than any other food. Meat is the only food that man can live on exclusively for long periods of time, and still remain in good health. It can also be easily stored through drying, smoking, and salting. Storage of vegetable products is sometimes a harder proposition.

Improvisation

This aspect of my program may seem obvious and self-explanatory at this point. However, to improvise effectively, one must have the proper frame of mind. Train yourself to think in terms of improvisation. Mentally explore the possible uses for junk and other discarded materials that you have access to. There will be plenty of these materials around, if our society ever does go down the tubes. So don't waste your time and energy trying to weave cloth and make clay vessels, when you can salvage clothes and steel pots from any number of abandoned houses and stores.

You now should have a good idea of how my survival program differs from the purists'. Be assured that I have personally used the methods and devices covered in this book. For the past forty years, they have allowed me to live comfortably and cheaply, away from the bureaucrats and social misfits that are ruining the quality of life in this country.

Certainly quite a few readers will be skeptical of my claims. Others will refuse flatly to believe that modern man can pit himself alone against his environment with only basic tools—and win. So please move on to the next chapter, and read the well-documented story of Bill Moreland, "Wildman of the Clearwater." His incredible story, which is verifiable by U.S. Forestry officials, shows us all that it can be done.

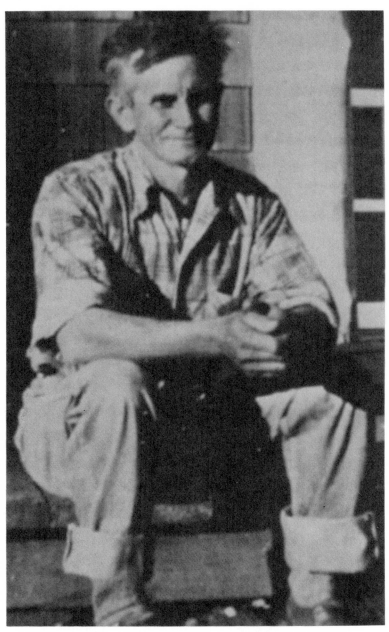

The only known photograph of Bill Moreland shortly after the Wildman's capture by crack U.S. forest rangers.

1. Wildman of the Clearwater

Sometime in the early fall of 1932, Bill Moreland headed for the mountains.

Moreland was, using a popular term of the day, a "ne'er do well." He had been born to an impoverished couple in Wolf County, Kentucky. At the age of three or four, his mother and father separated. Five years later, Moreland's mother died. At the age of eleven his grandmother, with whom he had gone to live, also passed away. Since Moreland's father was no longer around, the twelve-year-old lad was taken in by foster parents.

Unmanageable and wild, young Moreland eventually landed in reform school. From this early age, it became apparent that Moreland did not get along with other people too well. He continually ran away from his foster home.

The next few years sound much like a reform school travelogue. Moreland ran away, was caught by railroad police or a truant officer, and brought home, only to run away to such diverse places as Ohio, Texas, Wisconsin, and Michigan.

By hitching the rails and stowing away in freighters, Moreland eventually traveled over most of the United States. By the time he was thirty-two, he had split and loaded firewood, polished brass on a steamer, washed dishes, worked on a Coast Guard vessel, and mowed lawns. But mostly he was a plain old bum. Moreland also had many minor scrapes with the law.

Early in the summer of Bill Moreland's last year in civilization, he met a sheep rancher in Lewiston, Idaho. The rancher offered him a job on his ranch, located near the city of Mountain Home. It isn't clear how Bill managed to get to his new place of employment, but he did. Lewiston is in the North Idaho mountains. Mountain Home is, and was, a small community lying north of the Snake River at the edge of the Idaho desert, 350 miles to the south.

At least five days of hard travel on the best road in the most modern vehicle separated the two.

Moreland's past employment pattern held. He walked off the sheep ranching job forty-two days after he started it. Just why he left is not clear. Judging from subsequent events, Moreland probably slipped off under circumstances of interest to the "boys in blue." Perhaps it was a matter of "borrowed" supplies, advances on salary, or clothes and personal items bought on credit.

A Saga Begins

At any rate, Bill Moreland started walking—and walk he did. Straight north into some of the most rugged, treacherous, god-awful wild country in the forty-eight contiguous states. Today this same area includes three wilderness areas: the Selway, the Sawtooth, and the Idaho. There are virtually no roads there, not even dirt tracks. Even today, no cities larger than 100 people are found in this whole territory, and precious few places to resupply.

This didn't bother Wild Bill Moreland. He just didn't resupply. By his own admission, the Wildman talked to other humans only twice in the next thirteen years. He lived like a creature of the forest. Sometimes he stayed in back country Forest Service cabins or lookouts, but mostly the Wildman lived in hollow logs, in caves, or in holes dug back into hillsides and banks.

No certain record exists describing exactly what survival equipment Moreland had with him when his odyssey began. But we do know of a few things he didn't have, a compass and a gun being the most notable.

For the first two years the Wildman pushed steadily northward through the Central Idaho mountains. There was little big game. He lived on sage hens, blue grouse, ruffed grouse, and piney squirrels that he caught with snares, or knocked out of trees with rocks. Trout, whitefish, squawfish, salmon, and steelhead were plentiful in the creeks. If the game failed, there were always the Forest Service lookout towers with their emergency chop boxes— providing no warden was there at the time, and providing the snow wasn't too deep to get to the shelter. Forest Service lookouts are, after all, built on mountain tops where the looking is good, but the snow conditions are horrible.

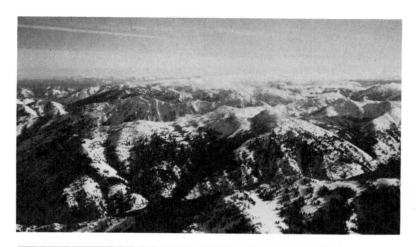

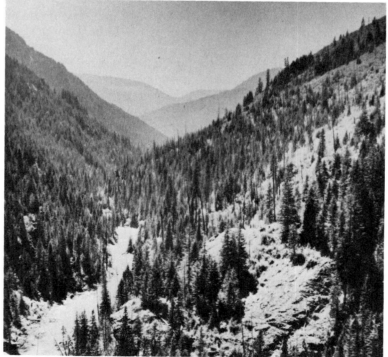

Top: Aerial view of the Sawtooth Mountains in Idaho.
Bottom: Lower fork of the Clearwater River, in the Clearwater National Forest.
This rugged territory was the Wildman's home for eleven years.

Another problem continually faced the Wildman. Since he was traveling on a line through the mountains, there was no opportunity to build up a series of food caches.

Twice during the first two winters, conditions became so grim that Moreland decided to give up and head to town. Each time he heard rifle fire as he approached civilization. It was only elk season in Idaho, but the mind-stupefying solitude clouded Moreland's judgment. He assumed the authorities were after him—the pattern that existed throughout most of his previous life.

The Clearwater

After two years of walking the Wildman reached an area north of Orofino, Idaho, known as the Clearwater National Forest. This nine-thousand-square-mile chunk of rocky crags, trees, mountain streams, and desolation became his home for the next eleven years. The Wildman stopped there principally because wild game was abundant. But as always, trouble and misery dogged his trail.

Often the passes and saddles drifted in with as much as fifty feet of snow. On level ground—such as it is in rough mountains—six to eight feet of snow accumulated every winter. First snows often came in September and did not melt away again until late May.

Some of the steep canyons provided shelter. Deer and elk migrated down into them to avoid the severe storms. On several occasions, before the Wildman made snowshoes, he was trapped by deep early snows.

He was forced to live for up to three months at a time in a hollow log, or under a bank, eating piney squirrels and martens. Often it was three to five days between meals of any kind.

After a few years, the Wildman learned. He built snowshoes and skis, cached food, stole clothing from Forest Service trail crews during the summer, and snared deer.

Still, the conditions were awful. His tent, when he used one, was a small piece of canvas draped over a rope. For years, Moreland used a rolled wool blanket for a sleeping bag. When he finally stole a regular bag from the Forest Service, he found his tent was too small. The bag hung out both ends and soaked through.

One time a bobcat stole his last bit of food, right off the fire. Another time he became horribly ill from eating raw frozen onions.

His poor diet rotted and loosened his teeth, so Moreland pulled them with a wire and bent sapling.

Moreland knew that his occasional thefts of food and clothing would alert and upset the Forest Service, so he avoided the regular traveled trails, walking the high ridges instead. This policy nearly ended in disaster during his earlier years in the Clearwater.

The episode started as Moreland was crossing a frozen talus slope high in the mountains, and he slipped. The Wildman slid and tumbled *several thousand feet* down the mountain on the slick ice. Bruised and cut, he finally stopped in a ten-foot snow bank, his pack, tent, food and blanket still above him, high on the mountain.

There was no question: if Moreland was to live, he would have to go back up the mountain after his supplies, through five feet of snow. He did, but it took him two full days to reach the meager little cache. In terms of enduring pain and suffering, this feat put Bill Moreland in a class by himself.

The Wildman's Capture

On 9 February 1945 Wild Bill Moreland's tragic saga came to an end. He was surprised in camp and placed under quasi-arrest by two crack Forest Service woodsmen. This climaxed a desperate six-day chase through deep snow in subzero weather.

At the time of his capture, Moreland was wearing a worn pair of field boots, covered by holey rubber pullovers. He had on an old pair of tin pants (naugahyde waterproof coveralls) and a mackinaw made from an old blanket. His captors were amazed that he wore no long underwear. The sweater he wore was stolen the previous summer from one of the rangers who brought him in. In his pockets the Wildman carried only a jackknife, fishing line and hooks, matches, and a bit of medicine (some bottles of clove oil and boric acid).

There was a Bull Durham pouch around Moreland's neck with a bottle inside. The bottle contained a homemade tin can key that the Wildman used to open Forest Service padlocks.

A few feet away a .22 caliber bolt-action rifle leaned against a tree. It had one shell in the magazine. Bill had a handful of spare .22 ammo in a small pouch. He had stolen the .22 and ammo from a camper in 1943.

1 0 *Live Off the Land*

His hat was obviously stolen. It came down around his ears. The Wildman's socks were actually dishtowels, which according to his captors "were wet and freezing."

Cooking utensils consisted of a small skillet and a coffee pot. Other than the previously mentioned sleeping bag, rope, and canvas, that was it. No mention is made of a slicker, belt knife, or ax, although the Wildman could have easily acquired one of the latter from almost any Forest Service cabin.

That was all the equipment Moreland had with him when his thirteen-year sojourn over some of the most rugged territory in North America ended. Even the Indians didn't try to live in the country Moreland called home!

Moreland as Teacher

So what does Bill Moreland's story have to do with living off the land in the city and country? Quite a bit, I feel. His true story should have tremendous impact on those of us who see personal survival as a primary concern.

Bill Moreland accomplished his amazing survival feat in relatively recent times. He was not one of the original legendary mountain men like Jeremiah Johnson, Bill Sublett, or Jed Smith who opened our country.

More importantly, Moreland did it in some of the worst country in the U.S., with an absolute minimum of equipment. Don't forget that he had no firearm of any kind till he stole the .22 in 1943, eleven years after he went into the wilderness.

The Wildman made it by existing very simply and by adapting whatever modern tools he could find to fit his particular needs. He didn't, for instance, refuse to use Forest Service telephone wire to snare deer, because he was into "pure" survival. This is an important point.

Just for the record, I am one of the most knowledgeable people left in this country regarding survival—that is, using wild edible outdoor products to live on. I have written an entire book on the subject of catching and collecting wild game, as well as innumerable magazine articles about similar topics. I have also given a number of seminars on the subject.

One thing is certain: most pure survival techniques either don't work, or lead to a life that is so miserable that few of us, myself included, would ever make it.

Pure vs. Practical

To live and thrive, the survivalist must realize that what he does and how he lives is going to have to be predicated on the basic thermodynamic law I mentioned earlier. Collecting wild edibles, providing clothing and shelter, and heating one's home must require less of your energy than you will gain back when the food is eaten and the firewood burned, and so on.

As the lines on a graph showing energy spent for energy received get closer and closer, the lifestyle represented by the graph becomes unnecessarily more uncomfortable. Bill Moreland is the best example of that.

On the plus side, lest we worry unduly about living in a hole in the ground as Moreland did, let me point out that most of us won't have to live in such rugged country, and most of us will have more modern tools to work with. Salvageable bricks, iron, wire, plywood, clothing, containers, and other materials will be all around us.

I feel my book will best serve the reader with a farm-kid mentality who has a put-it-together-with-baling-wire aptitude, not the pure esoteric survivalist who thinks our federal wilderness system is great because it would be fun to go live there after the collapse.

This book is dedicated to the truth that "pure" survival is bunk. It is impossible, improbable, and impractical. If you plan to make it with a crossbow, you will probably end up a corpse in short order. It's just that simple.

Just as Bill Moreland did, we must learn how to take the lumber company's phone line down and snare deer with it, or raid the figurative Forest Service cabin occasionally for an axe, a sleeping bag, or an item of food.

Millions of people won't make it either, because they lack the courage, determination, necessary appropriate skills, and/or foresight.

The places where you and I live are in some of the best environments for survival. They are locations where it was logical to build a city. When the time comes, even those of us who live in the country will be surrounded by a veritable wealth of useful materials. There will be an abundance of wild game, wild edible foods, and the opportunity to propagate more.

This books tells how to locate and use these resources, and how to collect them quickly and easily, avoiding a net calorie loss.

It is also a book about aesthetics. Many wild plants and animals may be edible, but they taste awful. Mature dandelions or raw ferns are good examples most people can relate to. Later on I will mention using common rats as a protein source. Obviously these things—dandelions and rats—are edible, but my intention is to stay away from these types of food. I mention them only as a last resort. We want to survive nicely in the best style our energies and intelligence will allow.

Our Future Roles

One last word of philosophy: When the time comes—and it will—we are going to have to revert back to being a nation of producers. There won't be any practical use for the OSHA inspector, land use planners, environmental activists, internal revenue agents, equal opportunity compliance officers, or the other millions of parasites in our society.

Everyone is going to have to be productively employed, thereby providing a needed service. Those who don't will surely fall by the wayside. To that end, I believe most of us who remain are going to have to operate on a barter system. I will want to trade some of my stored guns and ammo for needles, thread and cloth, for instance. Perhaps I will catch game for someone who will in turn cut and stack my wood. Garden produce may be traded for doctor's services, shoes for salt, and so on.

Each survivor will have to develop a marketable skill, plus have the tools and materials needed to use that skill. Those who don't are lost.

The coming crash is the best documented, most easily predicted event of its kind in history. No one can possibly say there was no warning. So let's get on with it and see how we can best survive the coming chaos.

2. Learning from Indians: The Nez Perce Story

Late in spring of the year 1804, a small band of Nez Perce Indians gathered in a camp on the south edge of the Clearwater River near what today is Kamiah, Idaho. Their camping place was at the far eastern border of their home territory. Two hundred miles of trackless wilderness lay between them and the Bitterroot Valley. Nothing—not even big game animals—lived in that wild region. They camped where they did for the purpose of waiting for the Lewis and Clark expedition to emerge from the intervening territory.

In retrospect, it was a good thing the Indians were there. Late spring snows and some of the most rugged country in North America were taking their toll. The Lewis and Clark party was on the verge of starvation and in desperate need of help.

The Nez Perce gladly provided that help. By Captain Clark's own admission, they proved to be the most unique and satisfactory friends encountered by the expedition on its entire three-year journey. The account of this meeting and the tribe's subsequent history are filled with lessons for the dedicated, practiced survivalist.

Although the Nez Perce had never seen a white man before the coming of Lewis and Clark, they knew at least six months in advance that the white men were on their way. Returning Nez Perce hunters apparently brought the news. No buffalo existed west of the mountains, so Nez Perce braves often traveled to Montana in search of these great shaggy beasts, or to participate in a little mercenary warfare on behalf of some of the less self-confident tribes. Opportunities to fight were extremely limited on the Indians' home turf. They amply proved the old adage that the toughest kid on the block seldom has to fight. Later when the Nez Perce led

13

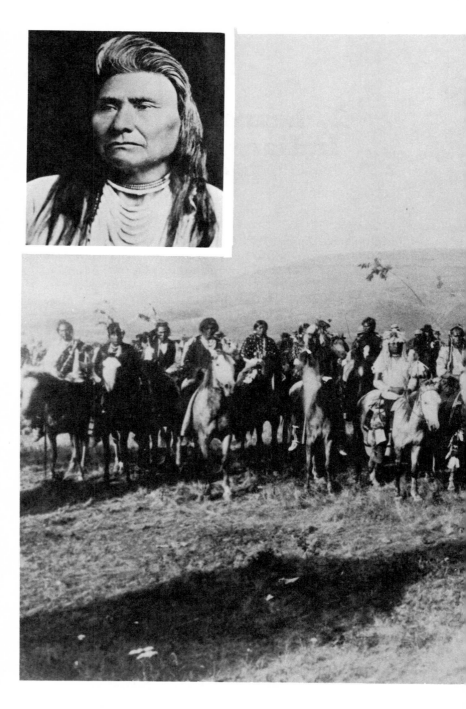

A group of Nez Perce braves astride their Appaloosas. During their war with the United States in 1877, they were described as military supermen. Their leader during this war, and ensuing flight to Canada, was Chief Joseph (*inset at left*).

by Chief Joseph battled the U.S. Cavalry, they were described by reporters covering the action as "military supermen," and indeed they were.

By the time the Nez Perce first met Lewis and Clark, they already had in their possession good workable firearms! What's more, in spite of the fact that no Nez Perce had ever laid eyes on a white man before, the Indians were reported to be extremely credible shots. The care and maintenance of their weapons was exemplary.

Certainly Lewis and Clark must have been surprised to see firearms in the hands of one of the most secluded, cut-off, unknown, little tribes of Indians they met during their three years' journey. But the mystery was not inexplicable. They soon learned that the Nez Perce picked up their weapons in barter deals with other Indians who had traded with the white man.

The Appaloosa Breed

Obviously any firearms in that place, during that time, had to have exceptional value. Something of equal or greater value had to be given in exchange, and in fact it was. The Nez Perce traded their beautiful, rugged war-horses for the weapons.

The Nez Perce first acquired horses about 1700, almost certainly from wild stock liberated when the Navajos went on the warpath, forty years earlier. Legend has it that one of their first horses was a white mare, heavy with foal. They watched her with great curiosity, and eventually became enamored with showy horses. In time, they bred exclusively for spotted or *Appaloosa* stock.

The remarkable accomplishment here involved the fact that the Nez Perce were the *only* tribe of Indians ever to master the art of selective breeding and actually develop a breed of horses. The superiority of the Appaloosa horses became widely known. Eventually a brisk trade developed that made the tribe quite wealthy. This was in part made possible by the fact that the homeland of the Nez Perce was ideally suited for training and raising horses. Some individuals acquired vast herds. Captain Clark wrote about one chief who owned about fifteen hundred of these wonderful animals.

Later, in 1877, the Indians used their money to fight a war against the U.S. Calvary. Often they stopped at trading posts along their route to purchase ammunition. Reporters at the time claimed these red men had deposits in every bank in the Pacific Northwest!

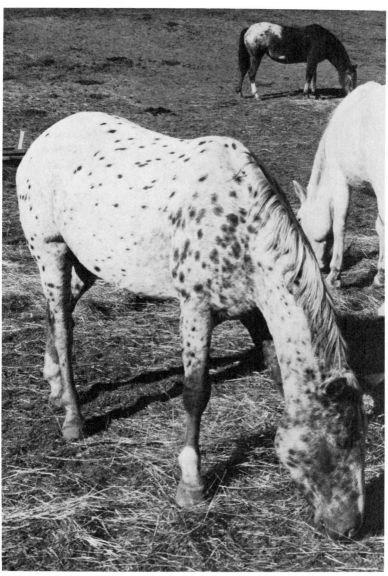

Appaloosa horses were originally bred by the Nez Perce Indians from animals lost by Spanish explorers. The Nez Perce were the only North American Indian tribe to perfect the process of selective breeding. These rugged, beautiful war-horses are the result of their efforts.

One old brave named Horse Tail was taken into custody after the tribe finally surrendered, with over six thousand dollars in gold coins tied on his belt.

Further Lessons

The Nez Perce domesticated cattle as well as horses, using similar castration techniques to upgrade their herds. As a result of all of this, plus an additional advantage or two, the Nez Perce were one of the few groups of Indians that did not have to periodically crowd together around a small winter fire and starve.

Each spring, they followed the moderating weather up out of the warm, sheltered canyons to the well-watered plains above. There they dug camas and cowish roots. Often, they collected enough in three days to last a year. Note that they dug carefully, nurturing the stock, so that it would grow back and be there next year.

As the weather continued to warm, the Nez Perce moved higher up into the mountains, where they caught blue grouse and fished for trout. Their large herds of stock thrived on the continually fresh expanses of new grass. In early fall, the Nez Perce reversed this pattern. They moved back down into sheltered canyons along the large rivers. Here were salmon, steelhead, and sturgeon as well as lesser fish for them to collect. Mule and white-tailed deer migrated with the Indians, who became expert at taking the animals for food.

In contrast to the Nez Perce, the American Indian, as a broad general class of people, relied first on domesticated plants as their principal source of food. After that they used—as they could—wild animals, wild plants, and then fish.

Domestic animals are estimated to have comprised less than 1 percent of the diet of the North American Indians.

Reliable records indicate that many Indian tribes would *never* eat fish under any circumstances, even though fish might be abundant. The Sioux preferred dying of starvation to changing their diet. When the buffalo were gone they would not eat beef, claiming it was too sweet. Other Indians preferred being on the dole to raising a garden. Their eating patterns were that ingrained and inflexible.

Compare this to the Nez Perce, who ate anything that was nutritious. In the final analysis, their greatest attribute was flexibility. These Indians were willing and able to adapt to their environment, even under bewildering and rapidly changing conditions. In so doing, they became a uniquely healthy tribe.

Lewis and Clark reported that the Nez Perce were the only Indians that were not interested in trading for beads, trinkets, and ribbons. They wanted awls, needles, pots and ax heads.

This adventuresome adaptability showed itself again in 1836. Five Nez Perce men retraced the route taken by the Lewis and Clark expedition, traveling on their own across America to see Captain Clark. Their plan was to see the now-retired explorer about the possibility of hiring reading and writing teachers to come back and instruct the tribe.

The Lewis and Clark expedition was a remarkable bit of exploring and adventure. The Nez Perce reversal was a genuine miracle. They found Clark retired and living in St. Louis. After a few years they did manage to bring back a teacher.

Nez Perce Specialization

Not only were the Nez Perce very adaptable, they were able to specialize in an area for which there was a demand, i.e., breeding Appaloosa horses. Experts in American Indian anthropology estimate that virtually every Indian in North America when Columbus arrived was either a part-time or full-time specialist. Contrary to popular but very misinformed opinion, the Indians did not generally roam around doing whatever. They were specialists—either hunters, skinners, clothes washers, animal tenders, or warrior police, to name just a few.

The moral here is that you and I, the survivors, no matter who we are or what we presently do, are going to have to adopt a similar pattern. We are going to have to be at least a part-time specialist doing something of value.

The Nez Perce, like the other Indians in North America, relied heavily on domestic plants for food. They did not rely on one supply of anything. Each year they put up a twelve-month supply of camas roots, being sure to leave the camas beds in good shape for the following year. Their care of the camas was likened by early settlers to a form of semidomestication.

Of course the availability of a given food source, and the ability to collect and process it was very important. It is also apparent that the Nez Perce had access to many natural resources. The important thing is that they learned how to use all of them. Then assuming that in the long run that might not be enough, they bred their cattle herds and nurtured their camas patches. It was a winning combination that made the Nez Perce uniquely independent.

To a certain extent, all Indians learned to use the things they found in nature about them. In some cases, it must have been a painfully lengthy process. Learning how to prepare poisonous acorns is an excellent example. Also, reliable techniques for taking game animals in sufficient quantities to live on are not developed overnight. Most of the ones we have today are ancient methods that have been refined and perfected down through the centuries. But now we are in real danger of losing all of them, as people sever and forget their ties to the land.

Learning from Indians

My strong recommendation to you is, as part of your survival preparation, to get out and research the Indian tribes that formerly lived off the land in your area, or the area of your retreat. Find out how they lived, what they ate, and if possible, how they collected their staple food products.

Research native crops to determine what grows in your area. Perhaps some of these might still be found wild. In most cases it will be better to lay away modern hybrid seeds, but at least let that decision be by conscious choice rather than necessity.

Quite a few Indian tribes subsisted on acorns. Oak trees are native to much of the U.S. Each year they produce tons of acorns, but most of the nuts are unpalatable or poisonous. Tannic acid in the meat gives a foul, bitter taste in small quantities. Some acorns have so much tannic acid that eating them, assuming one forces them down, would be fatal.

How did the Indians handle this? They learned that they could leach the water-soluble acid out of the pulverized nuts. The meal that remained made tasty mush or bread.

No doubt, the trial and error process by which they learned how to use acorns for food cost hundreds of lives. Trial and error will be necessary again, but not for the dedicated survivalist who reads and heeds. Previous study of the indigenous local Indian groups will go a long way toward obviating the need for such human guinea pigs.

Before leaving the subject of little acorns and mighty oaks, take note of the mention of tannic acid. Uses for this valuable material will be covered in the chapter on tanning skins.

One aspect of Indian culture that is very important, but which is lost in most modern societies, is the total use many tribes made of domestic dogs.

I for one am making specific plans to keep my dogs alive and healthy after the collapse. These include caching food for them, as well as medicine, leashes, and collars. It is important to me that my dogs stay alive and healthy for a variety of reasons.

Probably of first importance—I am going to need my dogs to protect my family and my property. No question but that there will be an immense amount of shooting, looting, and plundering. Conventional alarm systems will be worthless in the city. In the country, one simply has too much territory to guard. It would be virtually impossible under either circumstance to protect one's retreat without at least one dog.

A second good use for dogs is to find game. An Airedale, for instance, is a good watch dog. It will also point birds, retrieve grouse, tree squirrels and coons, and track deer. Other dogs such as Labradors and even beagles have a similar range of talents.

Under these circumstances, a good alarm dog would be a net producer of calories, but there is more. Domestic dogs are edible. Rather than killing the pups or neutering the adults, the owner can easily raise them for slaughter.

I realize this may sound nauseating and cruel. But in my estimation, raising hounds for protection, hunting, and food is far more realistic and practical than digging cattails for vegetables and killing snakes for meat.

Some seemingly logical sources of wild food may not appear to be available today. But wait. According to research I did on the Potawatomi Indians, a tribe that lived in the same country I did in Illinois, freshwater clams made up a good portion of their diet. But no one I know ever heard of clams in the local rivers. I just assumed that although the Indians ate them, overzealous clam-diggers and pollution probably depleted their numbers. I was wrong. Three of us went out one afternoon and collected a bushel of them. They were a bit strong but very edible. We boiled them thoroughly, since the river we took them from was somewhat polluted. Hepatitis is something the Potawatomis probably did not have to contend with.

My recommendation? If the literature suggests the Indians used a particular product, get out in the field and verify its availability. You may be pleasantly surprised.

At this point, people living in the plains states like to ask me how to go about building a buffalo trap. I have never killed a buffalo and probably never will. Not that it would be unduly difficult. But neither did most Indians. According to good solid anthropological data, white-tailed deer were the most common nondomestic source of protein for the red men in North America. Deer still live in every state in the union, and are reported to be present in double their pre-Columbus numbers. Rather than worrying about buffalo, these folks had better learn efficient deer-catching methods, some of which can be learned from the Indians.

Another lesson to be learned from the Indians concerns proper preparation of wild food items. Certain tribes ate raw meat and/or raw animal intestines. By so doing, they were spared vitamin deficiencies that were common in other tribes. Fish liver, for instance, is abundant with large amounts of vitamins A, D, B-1 and B-12. Vitamin C is found in raw meat, but it is destroyed by overcooking. This is the best reason for developing a taste for rare meat.

Habitation patterns today are basically the same as they were in 1492. This does not mean that there were similar numbers of people living in North America when Columbus got here, only that wherever people live now, they lived then. Wherever there were many, chances are that now there are also many. Where few existed, few probably live today.

By studying the Indians, the dedicated survivalist can get some idea of how many people the land will support. Probably this will be a very discouraging and sobering figure. Demographic experts estimate that there were about one million people here when Columbus hit the shores of Cuba.

Another question I like to ask is, "Did many of the Indians in my area starve to death around a fire of dried manure each winter?" If the answer is yes, I want to find out why and then make appropriate plans to see that it does not happen to me.

As a practical matter, each of us is going to have to survive and thrive wherever he is when society starts crumbling. The ambitious cut-and-paste innovator will make it, not the esoteric purist who is presently making plans to chew caribou hide in the wilderness of Alaska. The latter type of person won't even be able to get to Alaska, much less find a hide to chew.

Indians teach us which wild plants to use, but they also school us in the necessity of relying on domestic plants as well. We learn which wild animals can be collected and, more important than that, as in the case of the Nez Perce, that domestic animals can substantially improve the living standard of those who keep them.

Some Indians relied on one food source and suffered. The knowledgeable survivalist won't fall into that trap. As the Nez Perce did, they will have a domestic plant food source to supplement the wild plants they collect. They will learn to collect and use all of the game in their area, and then go out and develop domestic sources as much as possible.

Indians specialized. The successful survivor will have to do this as well.

Research Suggestions

Learning from the Indians is only one side of what may be as much as a six-sided die. It is a place to start for the guy who is going to make it in the wild and woolly world of the future.

How does one find out about such local Indians? Start with historic societies and chambers of commerce. One or the other may provide leads, assuming they do not have the information themselves.

City libraries or, even better, the libraries at state universities should have some good information. It is likely that someone has done research on your Indians. A call to your university anthropology department can turn up leads here. Check state and national forest service people. Often, park information officers are loaded with booklets and pamphlets. Some newspapers have people who can help. I would try the outdoor page editor, for instance.

Some readers may have Indian reservations nearby that they can visit, or they may know someone who has a working knowledge of Indian lore. My uncle was half-Ojibwa Indian. As a youngster, I learned a great number of outdoor tricks from him.

During my teen years, I met a man who was part Miami Indian; again, a good opportunity to learn that I took full advantage of.

If that fails, or is impossible, try the county agent's office. Often they know of people who have written histories of the area, or can provide other clues.

A very few hours of prior study will pay off big at the final hour. It may require no more than one evening normally spent watching TV. But the potential is tremendous for learning how to survive in one's own area.

3. Equipment and Caching

It does not take much equipment to stay alive, even under the worst circumstances. Bill Moreland proved that when he lived for over a decade in some of the most unhospitable country in North America, without even owning a gun.

But lest we glamorize Moreland, remember he led one of the most terrible existences that any man has ever known. He literally lived like an animal in dirt dens and hollow logs. The man was five-foot-two tall and weighed 130 pounds! He could fit into hollow logs. Some of us may not have that ability.

The first thing that the Wildman had to scrounge up was food. For the most part he lived off the land, but occasionally his situation became so desperate that he had to raid a cabin or Forest Service chop box.

The second items Moreland had to steal occasionally were clothing. To some extent apparel can be produced under pure survival conditions. In the long run, that may be necessary. Initially, I don't believe it will be, if some thought is given to the problem now.

Later, when he was interviewed, the Wildman claimed the most exciting thing he ever picked up was a .22 rifle. He managed somehow to live without a gun, but he lived much better with one.

Two other philosophical considerations and then we will move on to some practical suggestions.

Remember, the Nez Perce never starved. They developed more than one food source, and shaped their culture around domestic animals. This is one giant step farther than most other Indians went, who might have cultivated one crop, or raised horses or dogs, or relied on one source of wild game—buffalo for instance. But unlike the Nez Perce, other tribes seldom did all three.

The Cache

Throughout this chapter, I will be talking about caches. I believe caches are extremely important, as distinguished from the normal supply of goods and equipment that the survivor had better have handy in his home and/or retreat.

Caches contain supplies stored away in 100 percent secure circumstances, against the day of dire need. These supplies consist of the normal tools, food, and other items also stored at home for use after the collapse. Conceivably, I might not ever have to tap my caches, using instead the supplies already in my home and retreat.

If a person's home will also be his retreat as in my case, the needed supplies will always be handy. If your retreat is separate from your home, however, and there are questions about moving the necessary materials there, for God's sake plan on caching three stockpiles of survival goods.

Almost all of the goods I mention in this chapter are presently cheap. In three or four years they may be so expensive that you will weep at your stupid frugality for not laying away more of everything against the time of urgent need. Ax handles are a good example. Consider what they cost four years ago. Compare that to what they cost today, and then what you would pay if they were no longer available at all. About twenty years ago I whittled out an ax handle one winter. It took almost three months of spare time to get the job done! I have six or eight handles both underground and in my home supplies. Maul and ax heads, shovel heads, and pick heads will be easy to find. But the handles *will* be scarce.

I make my own permanently secured caches out of 6-inch ABS plastic sewer pipe. They are identical to the ones advertised in survival and outdoor magazines, which sell for sixty dollars or more. Even the homemade kind cost ten to twelve dollars. Keep in mind that it really is not feasible to cache unlimited supplies.

I protect home storage items by placing them in 3-gallon plastic buckets with seal-tight lids. We scrounge the buckets from restaurants, usually at no cost.

My rule of thumb is to store most items in these buckets. I save the cache tubes for things without which life would be all but impossible.

Begin construction of the cache tube by cutting a 4-foot length of 6-inch ABS pipe from the stock length. It comes in either 10- or 20-foot lengths. The 20-foot lengths divide evenly into five 4-foot cache tubes, but they are not always available.

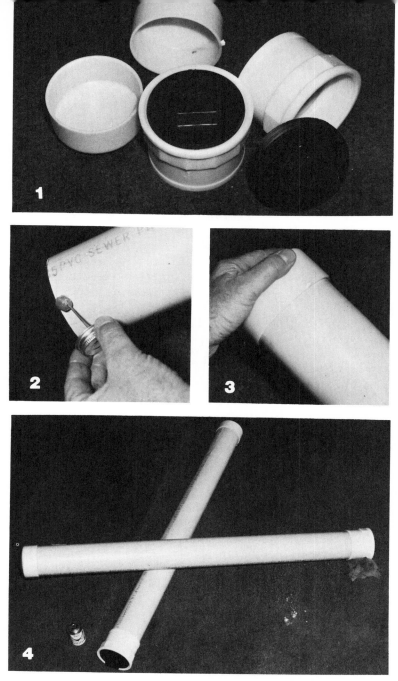

Construction of PVC cache tubes begins with cutting 4-foot lengths of pipe. (*1*) Each tube requires a permanent end cap, a threaded end cap, and screw-in plug. (*2*) Pipe dope is applied to the tube ends. (*3*) One cap of each type is placed on respective ends over dope and allowed to dry. (*4*) Two completed cache tubes.

Buy a clean-out adaptor and a threaded plug for each end of the pipe. Next coat the ends of the 6-inch pipe with ABS pipe dope, and fit the two clean-out adaptors on the pipe ends. In less than a minute the pipe dope will permanently set up. The plugs can now be screwed in place, completing the cache tube assembly.

As I said, at this writing a 6-inch ABS cache tube costs about twelve dollars to make. The finished result is without a doubt the best cache tube that can be had under any circumstances.

I have a number buried around my county. Although it may not be advisable, they can be hidden just about anyplace. One of mine is sunk three feet into the mud in a swamp. It has been there eleven years. The 5,000 rounds of 9mm ammo it contains are as bright and fresh as the day they went in.

Cache tubes can be made out of any size ABS plastic sewer pipe. For instance, 4-inch pipe is cheaper and easier to find, but holds a lot fewer goodies than the larger pipe. Some folks build special purpose cache tubes as small as 1½ inches in diameter by 18 inches long. These little tubes are sometimes used to store silver coins and gold.

Once in place, ABS pipe caches, no matter what the size, are hard to find. Long ago I planted one under a tree but neglectd to note exactly where. We tried to dig it up a couple of winters later, but had to give the project up. Later in spring when the ground thawed, I found it with a probe.

The easiest method of hiding a cache requires the use of an auger-type post hole digger. Drill a nice clean hole straight into the ground. Scatter any leftover dirt out of sight. Be clever about covering the cache hole itself. If the area is grass covered, cut out a divot of sod to fit over the hole. For cover, use leaves and brush in the woods, dirt in a flower bed, or whatever looks natural.

Should the cache contain items made of metal, take two precautions. If practical, put any metal objects in the bottom of the tube, then bury the top of the tube no less than 30 inches below the ground level. Deep burial like this foils the efforts of nosey authorities armed with metal detectors.

Be clever about where you put your caches. Readers who live in cities may feel their opportunities are more limited, but that is not necessarily true. Because of the presence of pipes, pilings, wires, reinforcing, and a host of other steel used to put a city together, it will be very hard to locate a cache hidden in the city, too.

Some suggested locations for urban caches include:
1. Arboretums
2. Flower beds
3. Under sidewalks
4. Small lakes
5. Marshes and swamps
6. Parks
7. Backyards
8. Parkways
9. Median strips between freeways
10. Gardens
11. In fence rows
12. Beneath houses in crawl spaces
13. Jogging paths
14. Gravel parking lots
15. Next to foundations

Be double darn sure to bury the cache deep enough so that it cannot possibly be detected.

Home Storage

I mentioned earlier in this chapter there are several reasons for having two types of caches: the 100 percent secure type buried in the ground, and the home storage types.

Home storage supplies are those I have laid away in my house over the years. By and large they are materials that I could get along without if my house was burned, bombed or looted. Materials in the buried caches are the ones that will be needed just to stay alive.

Most of my personal survival gear is the home storage type. This does not necessarily mean that your own cache system should be similarly oriented. Every reader will have to do a personal location analysis to determine what mix of methods is appropriate.

I live in a relatively safe, small city in the western U.S. There are no military targets within about fifty miles. The people hereabouts are conservative, self-reliant, and stable. When the crash comes, I doubt very seriously if there will be much looting, burning, or rioting.

On the other hand, we will be seriously affected by shortages of petroleum products, tires, manufactured goods, electricity, clothing, processed foods, glass, nails, spare parts, and ammunition, to name a few. In short, anything we cannot raise or that wears out will eventually become a scarce item.

Readers who live in cities will, I believe, be most fortunate in some regards. Because of the tremendous number of people who will expire, I believe that clothing will always be available, for instance. Parts for cars and trucks will be easy to scrounge from abandoned cars, which will be everywhere their owners used to be. There will always be some kind of shelter, and fuel to heat it in urban areas. The shelter may only be a boarded-up, gutted building that is heated with charred boards salvaged from surrounding structures. But this will be enough to keep the survivors inside alive. Making similar structures from scratch in the wilds, then cutting wood to heat it could be a life-sapping job, in terms of the energy exchange.

People in the country may be short of living space, if the exodus from the cities is as great as I think it will be. Food may not be as large a problem as it will be in the cities, but this will require planning and hard work on the part of the country dwellers. Obtaining fuel in small towns might also present a big problem.

Take the time to seriously evaluate your own situation. Determine what it will take to keep you and your family alive, based on where you will live or retreat to. Then decide how secure your survival supplies will be under the various plans I suggest. This is not something anyone else can do for you, unless you can afford to pay a high-priced professional survival consultant.

As I said, my home survival materials are all stored in the plastic containers commonly used by restaurants. These buckets have airtight lids and carrying handles, and are almost indestructible. The only drawback is their round shape, which wastes some space, depending on the items they hold.

These restaurant buckets originally contained salad dressing, fruit, cooking oil, and a host of other food products. Even a small restaurant will empty ten buckets in a week or so, and disposal of the buckets can be a problem for the restaurant. A few years back I started trading fresh watercress for our local cafe's discarded buckets. Now I have more than I need.

If restaurant buckets are not available, go to a discount store and buy some polyurethane wastebaskets with tight-fitting lids, and use these. Coat the lid with DuPont silicone caulk and screw it on

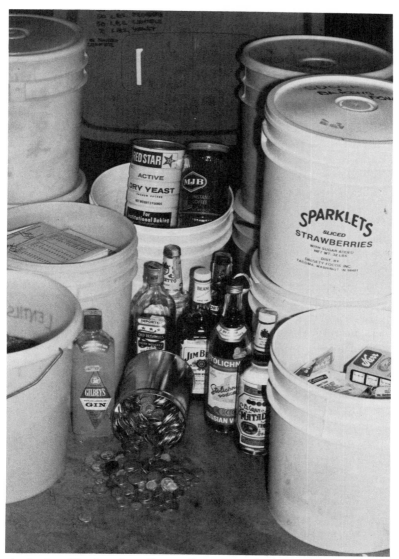

A selection of food products, liquor, silver coins, and other goodies stored by the author for survival purposes. All dried grains are stored in large plastic restaurant buckets, which are then sealed shut with screws and silicon caulking. Be certain to clearly label all containers in your survival supplies.

tight with ¾-inch number 6 metal screws. This will provide a fairly good airtight, varmint-proof seal.

Caching Survival Food

Some years back, I spent over a year in an extremely remote, primitive area in central Africa. It was not my intention to live a survivalist's existence when I went in, but that sure as hell is what happened. I literally had to scrounge everything I needed. When we were resupplied it was at two-month intervals, and then only with the most basic necessities.

As a result of that experience plus the many years I have spent living off the land in North America and other parts of the world, I have some peculiarities concerning survival stores that may not be showed by the purist. Here for your entertainment and consideration is my list. It should stimulate discussion.

The first thing I know I will need is something to eat. There is no way of knowing for sure, but I probably have a better ability to live off the land than almost anyone who will read this book. Nevertheless, an immediate supply of food is the single item I feel is most important to have readily available. These stored or cached grits should provide enough calories to give me, or you, enough time to start to live off the land.

So in one ABS pipe cache, I have stored fifty pounds of dried split peas to keep me going at the beginning, and that's all. One tube holds them all, safe and sound for at least fifteen more years.

At home, sealed in buckets, I have:

- 50 pounds of split peas
- 50 pounds of dried beans
- 50 pounds of flour
- 100 pounds of salt
- 50 pounds of sugar
- 150 pounds of dog food
- 10 pounds of coffee
- 25 pounds of rice
- 5 pounds of pepper
- 5 pounds of baking powder
- 5 pounds of baking soda
- 5 pounds of canned yeast

- 250 dried eggs
- 2 gallons of cooking oil

Old duffers who read this will recognize this list as being an old-timer's basic one-year grubstake. There is no salt pork or dried fruit, which was usually included in a grubstake. I intend to make these items myself. They spoil easily and are expensive so feel safe deleting them.

In addition, I try to keep both of our twenty-two-cubic-foot freezers at least two-thirds full of vegetables, fruit, berries, poultry, fish, and game all the time. Home-canned goods include stocks of pickles, relish, tomatoes, syrups, honey, and some fruit. We never touch the food in our survival stock. It is carefully stored in our basement, covered with heavy-gauge contractor's grade aluminum foil.

Food in our freezers and canned goods are used in rotation, but never, never depleted. We are always using but always replacing. One month we may freeze a bunch of ducks, the next a string of fat salmon, and a couple of deer the following month. In spring we may shoot a bear, grind the meat and render the lard.

The same is true of my root cellar. Several boxes of acorn squash may be there one month. By the following month the squash may have been eaten and replaced by potatoes, onions, or even hanging vines of tomatoes.

Several times recently we have calculated our food needs as compared to our food in storage. Assuming none of us would be able to snare a deer, trap a pheasant, or spear a fish, we would have enough eats for three full years. Just counting the dried food in our bucket storage, there is enough for almost one year for the five of us. This assumes the freezers quit and we are not able to salt, smoke, or dry their contents.

Although our food supply seems very adequate, it is what I feel my own family will need, knowing we will collect a lot of game, and raise a large garden. Other folks planning their survival cache supplies may want to lay by more salt, rice, or flour or add such things as macaroni and dried fruit. It may also be necessary to store a far greater percentage of this food in the underground cache tubes.

Also, some people may want to substitute dried beans for the split peas, do away with the rice, or make some other adjustments. I

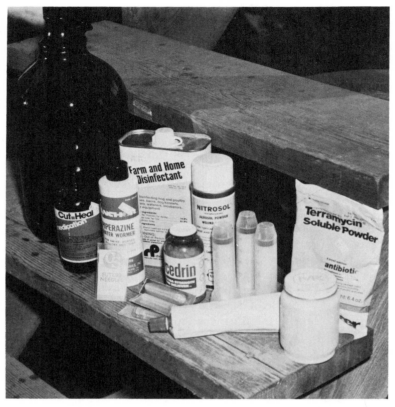

Veterinary-grade medical supplies obtained by the author through bartering. All items shown are suitable for human application, saving much trouble and money in the bargain. Depicted here are various disinfectants, piperazine for de-worming, suture needles and syringes, terramycin antibiotic powder, skin ointment, and some good old human pain-relief pills. Benson also suggests storing away birth control pills, or some other product with the same purpose.

Medical supplies of any type must be stored in a cool, dark place. Such climate control will extend the shelf life of the supplies, which can be prone to go bad after a few years. Periodically check expiration dates on all medicine for this reason.

like split peas and the last few years they have been ridiculously cheap.

Medical Supply Storage

The second level of needs involves health. Without a sound body and the resulting strong mind, survival is impossible. Wherever we traveled back in the bush in Africa, we were always treated like gods. Not because of our food or our equipment, but because of our gift of healing. Dozens of people lined up daily for the medical detail we supervised. They knew, and I found out, that one can miss a meal and live, but fail to treat a bad cut and it may be fatal.

Most of my medical supplies come from veterinarians' supply stores. They are cheaper, more available, and every bit as sanitary and useful as the human kind.

In my ABS cache, I have:

- 1 20-cc reusable syringe
- 1,000 cc's of disinfectant
- 1,000 cc's of antiseptic
- 500 grams of sulfa powder
- 20 terramycin tablets
- 5 #24 needles—1 inch
- 500 aspirin
- 1 large tube of burn medicine
- 500 birth control pills

Birth control pills or some means of performing their function are in a practical sense the most necessary medical supplies.

I always get a chuckle out of the tough-it-on-through survival epics one sees on the screen or reads in novels. The story line is invariably about a couple who walk from Shanghai to Paris. All of their companions fall prey to the pygmies, but by God they make it together, after only a few years of trying.

In real life, it doesn't always work that way. Many women who are not protected will have babies regularly. Survivors will find that to be a rough deal, especially initially. Other women will find birth control unnecessary as their systems shut down when lifestyles change and body fat decreases.

At home I have basically the same supplies, except for the addition of a small bottle of vet-grade penicillin that I keep in the refrigerator. Also, we keep a bottle of piprazine on hand, since internal parasites will be a problem in a survival situation. Most folks will need to lay away a supply of water purification tablets, bleach, or dissolved iodine. Our water will not be a problem so we have not cached that material.

I have a cooperative arrangement with a doctor who has his retreat up the road from ours. In return for his services, we have agreed to police his area and supply him with wild game—an example of that good old specialization that I said would be so important for the survivalist.

Caching Guns and Clothes

My experience indicates that the next two items are about equal in importance. Perhaps they both could be classified as protection. I am referring to guns and certain items of clothing.

There are four Stevens falling-block .22 caliber rimfire rifles and 6,000 rounds of ammunition in my seven pipe caches. All together, the four guns and ammo cost me about three hundred fifty dollars. After the crash I should be able to trade one rifle and 500 rounds of ammo for at least twice that much in value.

I favor the falling-block .22s because of my experience as a kid. There is little to go wrong with them. They will work fine even if a spring, for instance, gives out. They are accurate and inexpensive.

My cache also contains a military assault rifle of standard caliber and a large-bore pistol in a common caliber. There are 600 rounds of ammo for the rifle and 5,000 for the pistol. This may not be enough, but chances are good that my home cache where my main arsenal is will come through in good shape, and that will be sufficient. Rounding out this ABS cache are a belt knife, sharpening stone, and a gill net.

Most important in my clothes cache is a good pair of new leather boots for everyone. Putting these away was damned expensive but necessary, I feel. In addition, the tubes contain three pair of socks, two pair of long underwear, and a medium-weight wool jacket for each of my entire crew.

We have no special cache of clothes at home. All of us are very active outdoors. Our jackets, ponchos, shoes, and shirts are kept in good condition at all times.

Bill Moreland said the item he lacked most was something to sew with. I can second that—based on my many years in the bush.

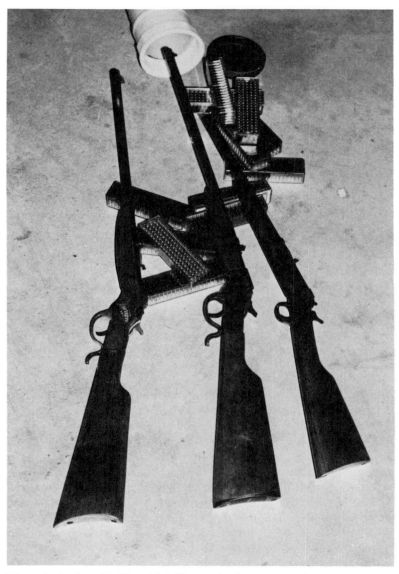

Three single-shot, .22 rifles with 1,200 rounds of ammo ready for caching. These accurate little rifles are inexpensive to buy, and are not prone to any mechanical failures. For the hoarder, these weapons are a good investment.

Setting aside a package of needles and a few spools of thread is minor, except in importance later on. We have these both at home and in the ground.

The Home Arsenal

In the next economy I intend to be an armorer, among other things. My list of firearms and related equipment is therefore not typical. I have put aside 40,000 rounds of assorted ammo, over seventy guns, a complete reloading setup, over fifty pounds of powder, thousands of bullets, and much more. I also have a half-ton of lead ingots, but these are for barter purposes.

For the average guy who wants a basic survival firearms package, I recommend starting with one accurate bolt action .22 caliber rifle with scope. If you already have one of these, lay away another. Store 2,000 rounds of .22 ammo in addition to those under the ground. Do not choose a lever action, semiautomatic, or pump .22. They break too easily.

Also store one good accurate bolt action hunting rifle complete with sling and scope. Do not take the open sights off, however. Put back at least three hundred rounds for this rifle. This may not sound like much, but you have to learn to make every shot count. When the chips are down, and if you do not try to blast everything in sight, the ammunition should last a long time.

I personally have no use for a shotgun in a survival situation, except for self-defense. The return on energy expended with a scattergun is poor. Birds will be taken with traps and snares. There will be no time for sport hunting. Most people have a shotgun already, so I recommend that they lay by two hundred to three hundred rounds of No. 4 buck to use to defend their retreat.

For most people, a pistol is a waste. Who reading this book would honestly admit that they could live off the game they could kill with one, even if ammunition was not a problem? The only good use I know of for a pistol is protection.

But better weapons exist for protection. I recommend one military assault rifle for each member of your family or retreat group. Our women have .223 caliber AR-15s. The men each have FN assault rifles in .308 caliber. To be practical, one should have at least five hundred rounds of ammo per rifle. Store more if you can.

Some folks include powder, primers, brass, and bullets in their survival supplies. This is recommended if you have reloading equipment and know how to use it.

Garden Supplies

The chapter on edible plants adequately covers gardens. Raising food is most important, but one must have the seeds to start with.

Most garden seeds keep a long time, and are very inexpensive. After determining what grows well in your area, buy enough seeds to store some underground and some with the home supplies.

Home Supplies

Here is a list of important sundry supplies to be stored at home or retreat:

- A white gas stove
- Single-mantle gas light, extra mantles and generators
- 6 gallons of white gas
- A down sleeping bag for each member
- A belt knife per person
- A large box of 4-mil plastic sheeting
- 250 feet of ⅜-inch nylon rope
- $5 worth of wooden kitchen matches
  Garden supplies should include:
- A rake per every four people.
- A shovel and hoe per every two people.

Heating Supplies

It is my contention that it will take a chain saw to collect enough wood to heat and cook with. I am afraid that without a power saw it will take six months to put up enough wood to serve five people, and we only live five hundred yards from the wood lot. Therefore, I suggest storing away two identical chain saws, a box of files, and an extra chain. I presently use the two chain saws I have, rather than keeping them in my set-aside stores. Obviously this is a risky procedure. I mitigate the exposure by keeping the saws in perfect condition at all times, and by never using the extra files or chains.

Also put aside a two-man hand saw with suitable sharpening file, and a maul, ax, wedges, and sharpening file. Many people

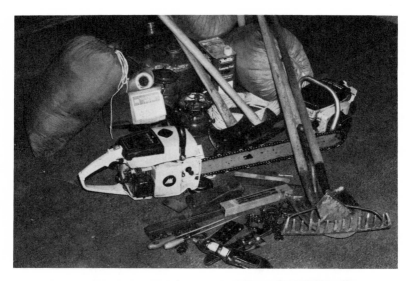

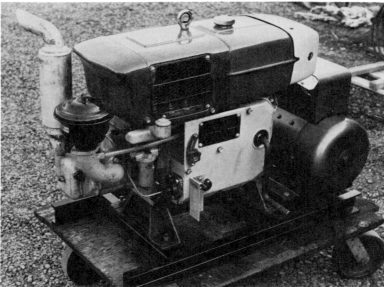

Top: A variety of garden and miscellaneous survival supplies. These includes tools, knives, lantern, sleeping bags, rake, shovel, axes, chain saws with extra chains, and a wedge for log-splitting.
Bottom: 12-horsepower Chinese diesel generator setup. (See later chapter on generators.)

tend to forget the necessary files to keep these tools going. Twenty dollars spent now will be worth five hundred dollars later when it becomes necessary to get an ax or saw back in shape, and nobody remembers how to make files.

And if you do not already have one, buy a small wood-burning stove that you can also cook on. Be sure to also put away the necessary lengths of stovepipe for the above.

If by chance I am caught in the city when the crash comes, I plan to heat with a small wood stove using old rubber tires for fuel. I will need to have a hacksaw and bolt cutter around to cut up the tires, and plenty of ventilation.

A very valuable item nobody thinks of—twenty bottles of good whiskey, if you can afford it, and are not tempted to use it prematurely. In three to five years the liquor will be quite valuable.

Maps

The survivalist who is going to make it in the country will need several good maps. Used properly, they can show where the game might be in the winter, where to find firewood, water, natural shelter, other people, no other people, access to an area, and so on.

The reason Bill Moreland pushed on through Idaho's mountains heading north to the Clearwater National Forest was because he had maps of the area. Apparently, the maps were inaccurate. Moreland is recorded as having some hellacious arguments over the location of terrain features with Forest Service people.

An extremely fine source of ground information that people seldom think about are pilot's sectionals. They cost a few dollars and cover more country in more accurate detail than most survivors will ever need. Buy pilot's sectionals at the general aviation terminal of your local airport.

Forest Service maps are available for most of the western U.S. and some of the East. Look up the nearest district ranger station in the phone book under the U.S. Department of Agriculture. Likewise, the parks services—both state and national—often sell maps. Most people live near one of these headquarters. Sometimes the maps are even free.

Bureau of Land Management offices have maps. It took me a while after I moved east again to realize most people in the U.S. think the BLM is a foreign car. If you know what they are, you know where to look for their offices.

Private map makers often sell their products through stationary shops and bookstores. Most are catalogued by county.

Military maps can be scrounged. Most people who live near military bases can develop contacts that allow them to pick up serviceable maps of the area.

County agents have aerial photos and maps of the area they serve. Sometimes the maps are a bit stale, but for the survivalist, they may do. Cost of an aerial photo is high. It takes an inordinate amount of time to get one made. But on the whole, when they finally arrive and are paid for, they are worthwhile, especially for the person who understands better with a photo than with a line drawing.

Bureaus of mines may have some very excellent topographical maps. Check at your state land grant college or in your capital city for the appropriate office. Some states have nothing. In others, the maps are outstanding.

Don't forget highway maps.

Maps are one of the little things that cost next to nothing now, but will be worth far more when the time comes.

Miscellaneous Suggestions

I have a 1,000-gallon underground fuel oil storage tank. With a little wood, I can heat my house and generate electricity for at least four years, using this fuel.

Keep gas tanks and reliable spare cans filled with extra fuel. Do you have a boat, for instance? The gas its tanks hold could run two chain saws for a couple of years.

A small electrical generator, as described in a following chapter, is very nice to have, too. Consider getting an electric welder to go with the generator, to do custom work with—again, the specialization factor.

If you opt for a generator, get a battery charger that will work on nickel-cadmium batteries as well. This way, flashlights, radios, and recorders can be kept running a bit longer. Don't forget a few extra flashlight bulbs.

Residents of both city and country locales should have a supply of steel game traps. It might even be wise to put half a dozen in your underground cache tubes.

Snare wire should be easy to find, no matter what the circumstance.

Whatever your job—tailor, baker, or candlestick maker—lay back the tools it will take to earn your way.

Things We Won't Need

This is not a complete list. It consists of a few items that many pure survivalists often recommend that I feel will be scroungeable or unnecessary. This whole area is one that is fun to contemplate, because sure as God made green apples, somebody is going to go out and start storing things like postage stamps, government bonds, and paper money. My list of "un-"necessities goes like this:

Pots and pans—Every house has some of these. With the population base greatly reduced, there will be plenty to go around.

Clothing—I just don't think there will even be one-quarter of the people left so we can use what the others leave behind.

Parts for cars—Stranded, ungassed cars will be everywhere. Scroungers will have a heyday picking up what they want from them.

Dollar bills—Need I say more?

Wire, nails, iron, fence, boards, hinges, and other raw building materials—These should be abundant in the cities. Gutted and abandoned buildings will provide all that anyone can use. City peple may want to trade these items to the folks out in the sticks.

I don't think we will ever have a particularly difficult time finding *ax or maul heads, chains, cables, shovel bottoms, rakes, and wedges.* Most of the tool heads I presently own came from abandoned home sites where I found them.

Caching and storing materials for survival is complex. Obviously the more that is put aside, the more comfortable one will be in the next economy. Well-equipped survivalists will not only be comfortable, they will be wealthy as well. What to store both underground and in one's home or retreat should be the subject of a great deal of thought and discussion. Hopefully this chapter will launch that process.

4. Locating Wild Game

Most practical survivalists will have to rely on some kind of wild game as a food source in order to make it through the collapse. Under some circumstances it may be possible to subsist on gardens, domestic animals, and/or barter, but I think this will be the tough way to go.

Many members of Indian tribes that relied on one basic food source starved to death each winter. As I mentioned in the Indian chapter, all of our native Americans raised crops of some sort. Some were hunters and gatherers as well. It was this mixture that really kept them alive during the unforgiving winters.

Collecting wild game alone did not generally work for the Indians, and it probably will not work for the survivalist. On the other hand, conditions are a bit different now than when the white man arrived.

In fact, I think it might even be easier to survive *now* via wild game collection. Archeologists and anthropologists give us good reason to believe that the principal meat protein food source for Indians as a class, was the white-tailed deer. According to estimates based on early records and current kill figures, there are more whitetails in North America now than in 1492. Some biologists think there are twice as many.

True enough, some species have been decimated. Buffalo are an example. But for your buffalo I will trade my European carp. Certainly there are more ponds of these in more different places available to more people in the U.S. than there ever were buffalo. In addition, we now have large populations of ringneck pheasants, Hungarian partridge, chukars, pigeons, possums, blackbirds, and dozens of different fish—all introduced species.

Also, realize that the competition for wild game is not nearly as intense today as it was then among the Indians. How many people do you know who can consistently go out and bag a deer? Or, who can gather ten or twelve rabbits and squirrels in an hour or so? Practically every Indian was an adept hunter. Today there are few people who are accomplished at hunting.

Our national orientation is directed at sport hunting and fishing. Under survival conditions it will be illogical and wasteful to wander through brush patches with a shotgun, or sit for hours with a hook and line waiting for a bluegill. Survival is too much hard work. There will be something important to do every minute of every day.

What few woodsmen still exist will mostly be programmed to try sport methods, and in doing so will tempt starvation. My contention is that before long, the practical survivalist will have the field pretty much to himself.

Those who will have to make it in the large cities will face a game-gathering situation different than the folks out in the country. The chapter on urban survival will cover semiwild game available to the city survivor.

Know the Game

My recommendation is that the serious survivor start developing his game-locating skills *now*. Take some long walks in the area where you will live during a disaster. Get used to finding game trails, tracks, dens, houses, and other animal signs. Practice all of this as often as possible to the point where you can locate game quickly and accurately. Make an inventory of your situation. List all of the outdoor assets available in your area. The game varies dramatically from one locale to another. Even within counties, a good population of a given animal may exist one place but not another.

Be aware that a surprising number of different game animals are either migrating or hibernating. In spring they may not be in the same place you saw them last fall. A few animals hibernate in the summer when it gets dry. Check all of this out before the situation is crucial.

Some game is difficult to collect, like mink, which are native to most of the U.S. The survivor can reasonably expect to run into them just about anyplace. They are moderately difficult to trap, especially for the beginner. Problems occur trying to use mink for anything. The skin is beautiful but is so small it hardly makes a good hatband. We cooked one up in a soup one time when we were kids. The finished product was horrible: stringy and strong. Thank God it made only a few cupfuls or we all would have been ill.

Emergency—Fish First

In a pure emergency situation, the first place I would look for a fast meal is in the water. Throughout North America there is a tremendous amount of fish protein that can easily be used as a quick food source.

"Fished-out" lakes and streams in your area probably contain huge populations of tiny, stunted bluegills, perch, or rock bass, and perhaps some fat carp. These fish have little sport fishing value so they are most often ignored. But they can make reasonably good eating. Their biggest problem can be preparation, which at times is a challenge.

Look in small farm ponds, sloughs, resort lakes, and other fairly small bodies of water. There are literally millions of these little impoundments in the Midwest and the South. Western ponds built for irrigation and erosion control often have similar populations of what are presently termed "trash" fish. While at these same ponds, keep a sharp lookout for giant bullfrogs and crayfish. If there are any frogs around, they will jump off the bank with a huge splash when alarmed. Frogs, over winter, crawl deep into the mud at the bottom of the pond. So if it's still early spring, don't necessarily conclude there are no frogs because you cannot see or hear them.

Big bullfrogs make a musical bass harrumping sound in spring. Sometimes they can be located by driving around the back roads on a warm evening with the car windows down.

Crayfish live in most streams in the U.S., but are sometimes hard to identify positively. Pond crayfish, on the other hand, dig vertical holes and leave a pile of dirt behind as evidence. These burrows are not visible in gravelly stream beds. In streams crayfish usually are found under large, flat rocks.

Supposedly polluted waters often support a thriving population of bullheads. These fish can live and breed in stagnant, tepid, silty water. Carp are often found in these waters too. Europeans eat these overgrown goldfish with relish. The lakes and streams of North

America support tons of carp, some weighing up to thirty pounds or more. Look wherever the water is deep enough to float a fish. There will probably be some. This is especially good to know about urban rivers, where carp may well be the only big fish available.

Other trash fish include the many varieties of suckers, redhorse, shiners, and minnows. These are all despised by the sport fisherman, but will be available in large quantities to the survivor.

Bass, pike, trout, perch, salmon, etcetera, are of course similarly available, if the competition is not too great. They can be taken with a limited amount of effort using the proper methods.

The training survivalist may want to set a fish trap or trot line to get an idea what the inventory might be.

Practically every place I have looked from Massachusetts to Texas and from Mazatlan to Valdez along the coast, there have been great numbers of saltwater fish available for harvest. Some are boney, small or supposedly taste bad. They do share one common trait—availability in quantity.

People who live near the ocean will probably have less problem collecting fish than those who will have to survive inland. Coast dwellers can also scare up other foods like clams, oysters, and crabs. You should start now to become familiar with collecting techniques for the fish/amphibian/crustacean-type critters for areas in which you plan to survive.

Turtles are a good source of food. In times past, people sought them out as a delicacy but now they are largely ignored. Some sea turtles are available to survivors along a gulf. Snappers provide the best eating inland.

Some sport fishermen have a general idea if there are turtles around. Asking those you know might be helpful. Snapping turtles are reclusive in nature and are seldom seen. The presence of mud turtles or leathernecks—both good eating themselves—is an indication that the bigger relatives are around. If you are not sure about turtles in your area, set a few lines and see what you catch, then practice cleaning and preparing them.

Ducks and Muskrat

While looking for turtles, check the swamps, backwaters, and bayous for other wildlife. Two good ones that come to mind are ducks and muskrats.

Most ducks are not permanent residents anyplace. They will fly either south or north every spring or fall. One cannot count on being able to use them as a food source all the time. Determine if the ducks in your area are there in winter, summer, or just pass through. Get a handle on how many might be attainable at what time.

Thankfully, muskrats don't take up and fly off twice each year. They can be identified in marshes by their grass houses, which look like miniature beaver lodges. There are also a lot of muskrats that live in burrows dug up under the banks of streams. The burrows look like underwater barn rat diggings. Black, dime-sized droppings and stripped willow twigs are other signs that muskrats are present around streams.

Muskrats, despite the name, are excellent eating. They can be caught in quantity, the skins used to make vests or gloves, and the flesh consumed with relish. They are definitely my favorite small game "eatin' critter."

Beavers and Coons

Beavers have proliferated to the point that many people feel they are more numerous than they have been for one hundred fifty years. Everybody knows about beaver dams, beaver lodges, and beaver-downed trees. Identifying them should be no problem. Get out and walk the streams and rivers.

The good old American beaver is an ideal animal for survivors. They are large, fairly easy to trap, and prolific. Beaver meat is reasonably good eating—not on a par with elk steak, but acceptable. And there is a lot of it. Some get up around eighty pounds. Beaver skins are warm, rugged, and large enough to do something with. Five make a good long winter coat.

Raccoons are another useful animal found around marshes, lakes, and streams. Experienced woodsmen look for scarred tree trunks that indicate a den tree. Less experienced outdoorsmen should search for tracks in the mud. The coon's front paw track looks a lot like a human hand. Coon live on berries, mice, fish, crayfish, fruit, corn, and other agricultural crops. They are found pretty well over the entire U.S., except in severe snow country.

During the winter, coons hibernate for weeks at a time. They stick their noses out on warm nights for a few hours, but that's all. During that time it is tough to catch them regularly.

Porkies

From the time the first colonists had landed, porcupines have been a mainstay of the survivalist's diet. When we were kids it was considered poor form to kill a porcupine in the deep woods.

"Some poor lost hunter may need the porky to live on," was the common saying. After a few years that changed. It became the in-plan to try and "keep the porcupines in check, 'cause they sure kill young pine trees."

Nowadays nobody thinks about porkies much any more. Apparently the pendulum stopped about in the middle.

Porkies are easy to chase down in the woods and do indeed make good survival rations. They are large—some weigh twenty-five pounds—and very tasty eating. The problem is finding them. Expert foresters and hunters are able to walk through a woods and determine if there are porkies around. They look for chewed limb ends, treetops, and dead trees. Younger trees are especially susceptible to porky's damage.

All of this is not immediately apparent to the novice, unless the population of porkies is approaching the lemming stage. You might try your luck at locating porky sign in the woods, or just be content to be in the woods till one crosses your path. In the snow, the trail is wide and pudgy. Look for marks from the large dragging tail.

Squirrels, Possums, and Rabbits

Food animals—those fairly low on the food chain—are always good bets for the survivor. Muskrats and porkies have already been mentioned. Others are squirrels, possums, and rabbits.

In my opinion it will only be worthwhile to hunt squirrels in town. Out in the country they are too wise. Hunting wild squirrels will produce a negative calorie flow. It might be possible to trap them, which of course is more efficient, but planning to sit under a tree with a gun and wait for them is not too smart.

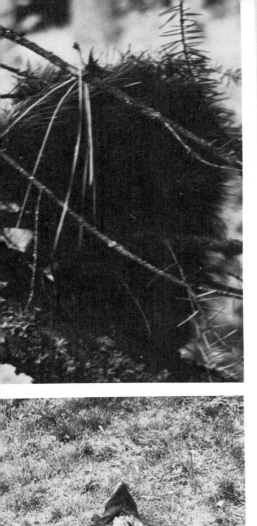
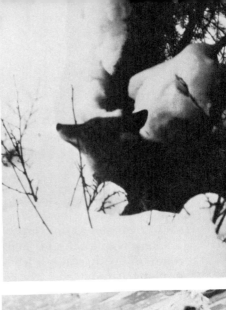
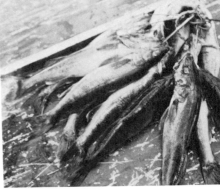
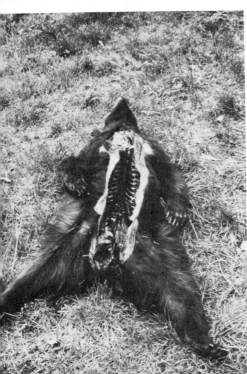
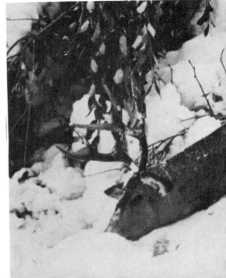

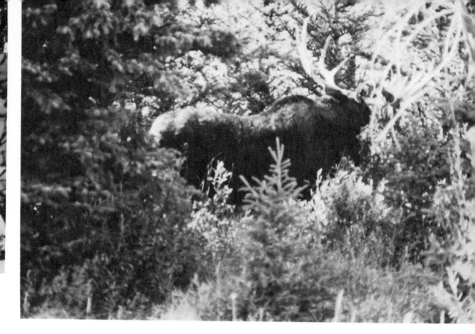

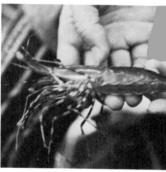

The selection of game open to the knowledgeable survivalist is indeed vast. Some types, like the walleyes at left, can be taken with only a piece of gill net and a good knowledge of the territory. *Clockwise from top left:* a treed porcupine, a coyote in winter; photograph of a moose in the bush; an ocean prawn taken in a trap off Mexico; a nice mess of salmon; an eleven-point mule deer; and a black bear "down on the grass" and ready for the skinning knife.

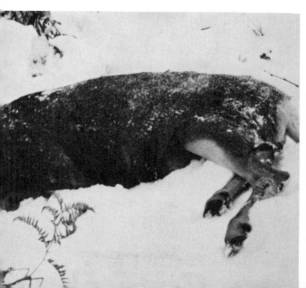

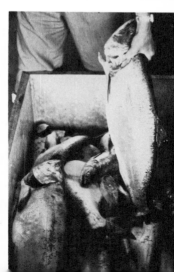

People who live in town already know if there are squirrels around. What they usually don't know is how many there are. I and my family have, for instance, collected numerous squirrels in a large city with no discernible impact on their population.

Out in the country the average squirrel is darn tough to see. Invariably they will spot you coming before you spot them. Leaf nests high in the trees or at the end of wild grape vines, chipped tree trunks, and cuttings under nut and fruit trees are all good indications that squirrels are present.

My recommendation for those who want to know if possums are around is to watch for road kills. In times past when there was more sanity and less money, the Fish and Game people used to estimate wildlife population levels on the basis of reported road kills. It was and is a good method of determining the population density of animals in an area.

Otherwise, possums are difficult to identify in the woods. They live on fruit, berries, nuts, mice, frogs, grubs, and to some extent domestic crops. Sometimes their odd, globular tracks can be seen in the mud. Possums have expanded their range up into northern snow country somewhat. Wherever they have migrated, they sleep a lot in the cold winter.

Catching possums in traps is easy, since they're awfully dumb. The skin is large enough to do something with. Possum lard makes excellent soap, and the meat is quite a delicacy. A big one weighs in around fifteen pounds so they are worth catching.

Rabbits or hares are everyplace in the U.S., except deep in the core of larger cities. Most people first see them standing around the edges of open areas in the morning and at dusk. Look for runs and burrows. Rabbits are not large, unless one runs into western jackrabbits. They don't hibernate so are available even during the worst winters.

Upland Game Birds

Other animals that reproduce rapidly and are good food for readers are the various upland game birds. Some places in our country, more of these birds die in the winter than are annually hunted.

During the spring and summer, pheasants and some kinds of quail can be heard calling. At other times of the year game birds will come to gravel roads to pick grit. At sunup or sunset they should be obvious, lined up like so many soldiers swallowing stones. If there are very many birds, your walks in the country should reveal the fact. Especially in the early fall, a bird or two should be flushed every quarter of a mile or less. Tracks in the snow are also good indications.

Turkeys are sometimes collectible, but often are not visible. Look in a wildlife book to determine if you or your retreat are in turkey country. If so, ask the farmers and ranchers in the area for specific locations. Many times no one but a few game department people will realize there are wild turkeys in a given place. You'll just have to root out the information for yourself. Trapping these animals is not difficult if the trap is set where turkeys are. Nice edible birds live throughout America. They range from three kinds of grouse to a whole range of quail, partridge, and pheasants. In the unlikely event you are ignorant as to what is available in your area, get a picture book and identify the wild fowl you saw standing along the road.

Deer

Taken as a whole, the North American Indian used deer as a protein source more often than anything else, probably because deer were and still are abundant and easy to catch. Give them eight trees and a dozen blades of grass on four acres and they will hide and proliferate.

Deer give themselves away in an area by beating down trails and making a lot of tracks. They hang around old orchards, maturing fields of grain, and, if you put one out, salt licks.

They like to hole up during a cold winter. When spring arrives, they come out and eat the tender new field grass. Fall is the time to find them in orchards and corn fields.

Most deer hunters fail to see more than 1 or 2 percent of the deer living in their area. Whitetails are a whole lot smarter than the average human who walks through the woods. As a rule, deer are less wary in the spring and early summer. Hikers often see them standing around fields early in the morning or at sunset. In the fall it is easy to do a private deer census. Drive the back roads after dark and shine a spotlight across open fields and into the woods. In four hours you will know virtually every deer concentration in the county. Just don't carry a rifle along in the car or police will nab you.

Salt licks will attract deer, but mostly only in the spring. Later on in the year, salt may hold them in the area, but it won't necessarily bring them in.

Given those parameters, a salt lick is a good investment. I suggest putting one at a point with fairly good visibility where several existing deer trails come together. It is better if some cover already exists near the lick so the deer will be less timid about hanging around. Brown or blue mineral salt is less conspicuous. Rock salt won't last as long as blocks, but is very hard for people to find, if establishing a lick might be a problem.

Get the salt out early. A salt station that will attract and hold game takes about two years to become established. Clay soil holds salt better. The game will eat the ground after the salt has dissolved.

Big Game

Common old black bears will be a viable food and product source for the survivor. Happily it has been my experience that there are more bears around than most people suspect.

I have gotten them within an hour's drive of Denver, Seattle, Minneapolis, and Detroit. These animals, however, are like mist in the woods. They can drift through without you ever knowing they are there.

Bears give themselves away by crapping in the woods—no kidding. Look for large piles with berries, bugs, and grass. If no paper is near, it's a bear. Pad marks in dusty or muddy trails are other good evidence.

I usually decide how many bears are in an area after looking at the old rotten logs and stumps. If they are badly torn apart there are many bears.

Moose and elk are often so wide-ranging and evasive that getting one will produce a net energy loss, even given their large size.

Many animals are either too hard to take, provide too little usable product, or taste terrible. Coyotes, fox, marten, and badger are good examples of these.

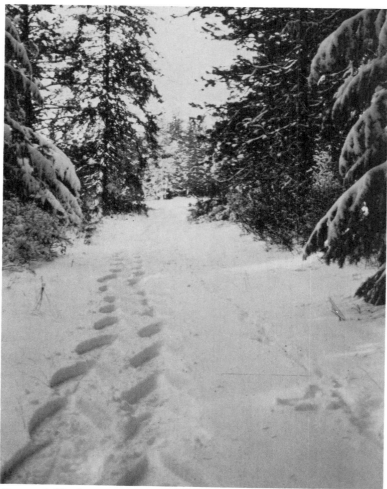

Deer tracks like the ones shown on the right are easy to spot in the snow. In case you haven't guessed, human tracks in the snow are shown on left. Because of this type of disturbance, Benson feels it is best to construct deer snares before the first snowfall of the winter. Otherwise the snare set will be surrounded by a mess which reeks of human scent.

Obviously there is a lot of wild edible game out there. This chapter does not provide a complete list by any means, but it should serve to sensitize readers. Start now by taking long walks in your area. Practice till you can locate game quickly.

Finding game is a lost art for most Americans. It's also an essential business for those of us who are going to survive.

5. Snares and Deadfalls

Before the coming of the white man, the only traps Indians had to use were rough, jury-rigged affairs that either fell on the animal and killed it, or lassooed it.

Since most Indians didn't fool around catching small game to any great extent, the above fact shouldn't be overly impressive. The Chippewa Indians, for instance, occasionally trapped beaver and otter, which were plentiful in their home territory. The pelts they did take were more decorative than functional. Often the animals were killed in the spring or summer when it was easiest to accomplish. The fur was, of course, not prime. It had very little wearing value.

Europeans interested in furs for warmth and beauty stimulated an interest in small game which in turn encouraged the Indians to set more traps. Early traders reported that it was quite a chore to get the Indians to trap during the winter when the pelts were prime. Along with their interest in fur, the white men brought in two items that allowed for expansion and improvement in the art of Indian trapping. These were brass wire—used for snares—and iron ax heads. The axes made construction of deadfalls many times easier. It now became practical to cut and shape wood quickly and easily—necessary technology if very many deadfalls were to be built.

Modern day woodsmen will certainly agree that if all it takes is some wire and an ax to make it in the world of a crashed economy, it might be possible to survive. I, for instance, believe that if we don't produce another new piece of wire for the next ten years, I will still be able to find enough lying around for all of my needs.

The stinger here is not finding the raw materials, or even locating the game. The problem will be learning how to catch the game in primitive, homemade traps. It took me about five years to become proficient with snares. I have been fooling around with deadfalls for more than forty years, and truly believe I could still do much better with them. Any outdoorsman left in the U.S. who knows how to build a deadfall almost certainly learned how as a farm kid during the depression. At the time it was virtually impossible to come up with the thirty-five cents needed to buy a steel trap. People like me had to make do.

Yes, conditions were pretty tough during the last depression. Yet there will be an even greater incentive during the next collapse. One's line of primitive traps may be feeding the family.

I recommend that you start today learning how to use snares and deadfalls. Build a few to see how well you can do with them. Maybe some harmless practice on your pet cat would be appropriate, or if you live in the suburbs, animals as common as starlings and grackles will do.

Take some trips out in the country in the vicinity of your intended retreat. Evaluate the wild game inventory, both in and out of the city, and try to determine its susceptibility to the use of snares and deadfalls.

Deer are probably the easiest animals to snare. Any creature that follows a regular, well-defined trail, pushes through brush, and walks with its head forward off the ground, can be snared. Deer fall very nicely into all these categories. Rabbits are an easy-to-snare animal. Not only do they possess the required traits, they are exceedingly abundant. Nutria are another fairly good eating animal that are easily caught in snares. If you live where nutria do, include them in your inventory.

There are literally hundreds of trap variations based on the use of snares. If, after reading this chapter, you start to come up with other variations of your own, rest assured. You are on the right track and probably can survive by taking game with snares.

Making a Small-Game Snare

The quick, easy method of making a simple snare is to use standard appliance wire. These little numbers are cheap and easy. They provide a nice start in the snaring business.

Cut a piece of standard number 16 electric cord into 20-inch lengths. Split the two rubber-insulated parts and strip the insulation off the wire. Discard the old insulation.

Before continuing, check the resulting bunch of hair-thin copper wires to be sure they are fresh enough to be bright and malleable. I have, in years past, caught a few fox using a solid copper wire snare. Generally they break or untwist the solid wire, so I don't recommend it for fox. Leave the wires in their present thickness without further division if you plan on snaring fox. Otherwise, start splitting the bundle of wires in two equal parts.

This untwisting may be a bit of a problem if the bundle is heavily intertwined. Keep working at it till you have a bundle of about 12 hair-thin copper wire strands remaining.

Twist the ends into small end loops and pull the main line through, forming a lassoo. Copper wire is malleable enough to retain its shape on its own. It will hold the loop and then snare smaller game without a locking mechanism. The result is a basic snare that can be used in dozens of different situations.

Make a loop about the size of a teacup for rabbits, and set 3 inches off the ground in a well-used run. Tie the wire to a small bush that is strong enough to restrain a struggling hare. The best time to snare rabbits is in the winter when the runs are obvious in the snow.

A few pieces of grass placed in front of the snare will hide the wire and encourage the rabbit to push through into the loop. By so doing, it will cinch itself into the snare more tightly than if there were no obstacles. Similarly, wire snares work very nicely at entrances to dens. I put the snare in the hole and then cover lightly with leaves and grass. Groundhogs, for instance, will push out through the plug, hopelessly fouling themselves in the wire.

Snare Variants for Small Game

A good variation with these simple snares is to set them up in trees for squirrels. Food trees, such as ironweed, hickory, and buckeye, are good bets. In the short run, squirrels will tend to sit and eat in the same places in trees, or as the hillbillies call it, *cutting.* Look under trees for piles of hulls and shells. Determine which branch they probably sat on and how they got there. Then it is an easy matter to put two or three snares on the limb.

Unless you have huge squirrels, the snare loop should be 2 inches in diameter or even a bit less. Staple the end of the wire to the limb and set so the bottom of the loop is about 1 inch above the limb. I always set these snares horizontally, although some of my

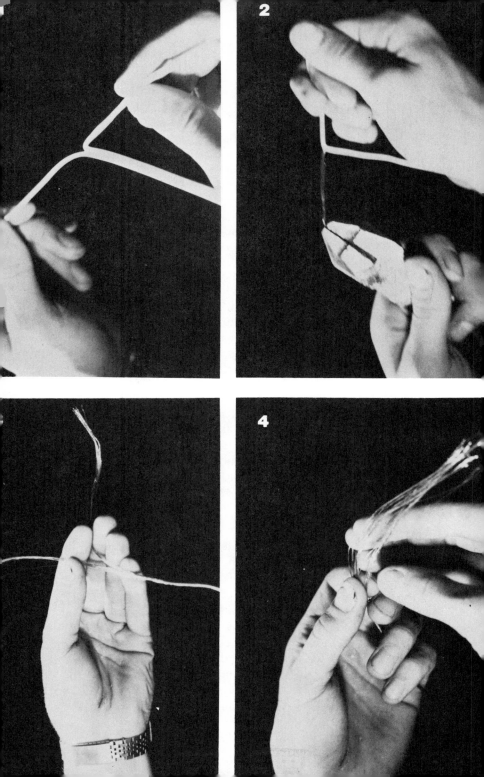

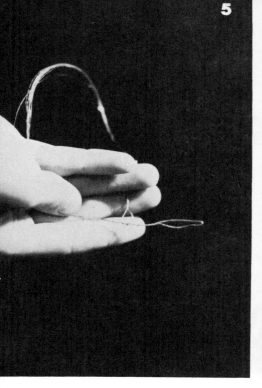

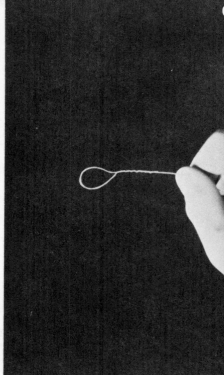

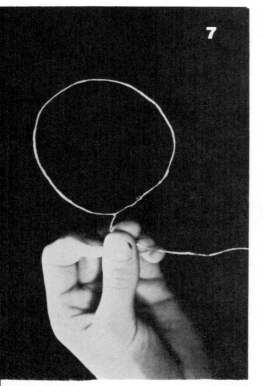

Technique for making a wire small game snare from common appliance wire. (*1*) Split the two insulated halves of the appliance wire or cord. (*2*) Pull the wire free of the insulation. Be sure the pliers grip all wire evenly. (*3*) Unravel the exposed wire into two even bundles. (*4*) Continue unraveling each bundle into groups of 12 hair-thin wires. (*5*) Twist the 12 wires into a single strand. Length will be from 12 to 20 inches, depending on intended game. (*6*) Small loops are twisted into each end of the wire. One becomes part of the main snare loop. An extra line can be tied to the other small end loop, depending on use. (*7*) The finished snare. Note the small end loop contained in the snare lasso is pulled tight.

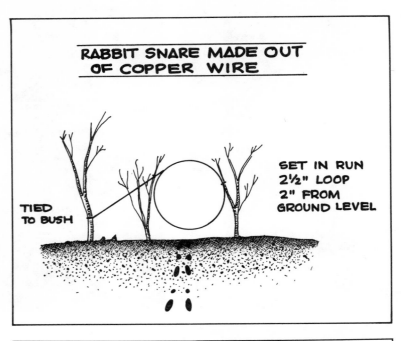

RABBIT SNARE MADE OUT OF COPPER WIRE

TIED TO BUSH

SET IN RUN 2½" LOOP 2" FROM GROUND LEVEL

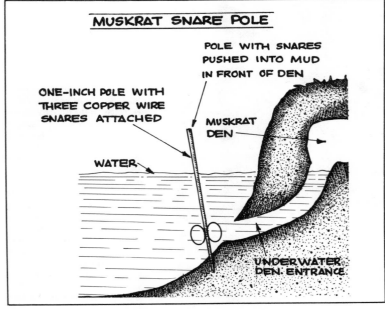

MUSKRAT SNARE POLE

POLE WITH SNARES PUSHED INTO MUD IN FRONT OF DEN

ONE-INCH POLE WITH THREE COPPER WIRE SNARES ATTACHED

MUSKRAT DEN

WATER

UNDERWATER DEN ENTRANCE

friends claim they catch squirrels in vertical loops nailed to tree trunks.

Muskrats are another type of small game that can be taken nicely with copper wire snares. One of the best techniques is to rig two or three loops on a solid 1-inch pole. Place the snares on the pole about a foot from its end, and push the other end into the bottom of the pond where the muskrats live. The snares should stand out in a fashion that will guard the underwater approaches to the muskrat dens. When the rat swims by, the snare should be in a place where it will encircle it.

The best way to capture the average ominvore like a fox, coyote, or even a coon or possum is to use a large bait. A dead cow, deer, or sheep is ideal. Set a snare or two in each trail leading to the bait. Some of the snares can be as much as fifty feet away.

My favorite beaver set, after the ice is on, involves using snares on a cedar pole. Staple three or four branches of fresh aspen on a 3-inch dried pole. The aspen is the bait. String at least one snare per foot on the pole. Push the pole into the mud in the bottom of the pond and pack snow around the ice hole.

Beavers hungry for a fresh log to chew will circle the pole. Eventually they tangle in the loops and drown. The outfits are not very efficient which, under the circumstances, is not important.

Snaring Birds

Birds, especially game birds in the pheasant/grouse/quail category, are relatively easy to take with snares. Use a thin 6-strand snare in winter in the bird's run. Sometimes it works well to set three to six snares in a gang around a handful of corn or wheat bait. This method is very effective when the birds finally start working the bait continuously. Usually this happens late in the season when other food has been consumed.

Sparrows, robins, pigeons—any birds—can be taken in the city with snares, if the snare can be set where the birds land. Sometimes finding the place where these birds roost can be a real chore.

Snaring Fish

My first use of copper wire snares as a kid was for catching suckers and carp out of a river. Sometimes, if the fish were docile and we were especially sneaky, we could get them with nothing

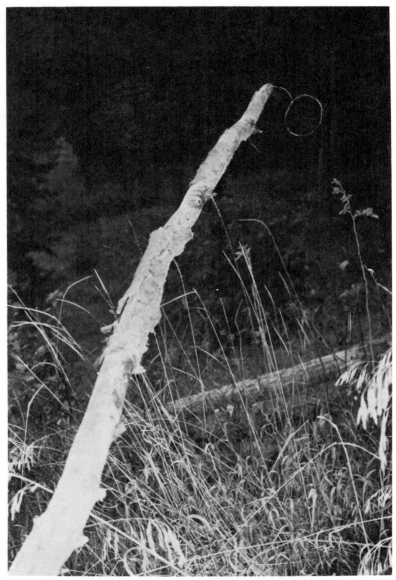

Pole rigged with wire snare loop on one end is placed over area where game birds are feeding. This trick works particularly well where the birds are feeding on "nits," or newly-hatched flies.

more than a 5-foot wire with a snare loop on one end. However, it is easier to find a nice springy 10-foot pole (cane is ideal), and attach a copper wire snare loop to one end.

In order for this method to work, you must be able to see the target fish cruising without being seen yourself. Stand back from the water's edge as far as possible. All of this may take a good deal of judicious sneaking around.

Loosen the snare up so the loop is about twice the size of your intended catch. Hang the snare in the water, maneuvering it around till the fish starts to swim through. Give the rig a sharp jerk. If your timing is right, the snare will dig into the fish right behind the gill cover. Even a snare cinched elsewhere on the body should hold if the initial jerk is sharp. Again, the copper wire will cinch tight and stay that way, holding the fish for you to pull out of the drink.

Very small fish are difficult to collect with this method. Fish over six pounds can be tricky to pull out of the water, since their weight can break the wire. Twenty- to thirty-pound line is needed here between the wire loop and the pole.

Snaring is especially effective in reefs and jetties for ocean fish such as sea bass, mackerel, grouper, and sharks. Almost any fish that can be seen can be snared.

Big Game Snares

Larger game can be taken with snares but, of course, the snare has to be proportionately heavier and more complex. Be warned, though, that most people I have seen make their snares out of wire or cable that is too heavy. The result is a rig that is too inflexible to get the job done.

I often use light airplane cable to make my large snares. In some places in North America it is still possible to buy snare cable, or you can use TV antenna cable, guy wire, telephone wire, old automobile cable; even baling wire, barbwire, fence wire, or solid copper wire can be made to work in a pinch.

There are two additional parts to a larger, more sophisticated snare that survivors must consider. Either part can be constructed at home, or made from existing materials.

Remember that our small, copper wire snares rely on the ductile nature of the wire itself to stay cinched tight. Heavier cable snares

require locks to achieve this. I make my locks out of pieces of
L-shaped iron, with slightly oversize holes drilled through each
arm of the L. Loop one end of the cable through one L hole,
and fasten the cable end to the other L hole with a crushed nut or
cable clamp. The V in the L lock should point to the center of
the loop for best results.

Some snares, especially those used on very large animals, should
have swivels built into them, which is the second consideration.
Without swivels, the animal will often twist the wire beyond reuse.
Often this will happen even with swivels. I buy small steel-rope
swivels, or even large fishing swivels, for use on my snares. The
swivel is attached between the snare loop and the main length of
cable.

Coyote-sized animals are best taken with 1/16-inch cable snares.
Many times, snares will work much better for these animals than
steel traps, because they won't freeze up. The cable should be 3 feet
long.

Deer snares are generally made out of 3/32- or 1/4-inch cable.
Many times, heavier cable will work just as well. Venison stew is so
easy to acquire with a snare, that you will wonder why in the world
a survivor would ever wander around the woods with a rifle looking for them.

There is considerable difference of opinion regarding the actual
in-field use of a deer snare, which can take many forms. I like to
cinch a nut on the cable of my snares, which is stopped by the lock.
The nut then serves to keep the deer from strangling itself. My
brother, for example, wants his deer dead as soon as possible. They
don't beat themselves up too much, but I don't like to eat strangled
venison. Brother advocates using a bell on the snare to broadcast
the fact that a critter is in the trap. But I am not sure I want to
broadcast the location of my food to the whole world.

I make my deer snares about 7 feet long. The additional length is
needed on deer snares so a spring pole can be used. Good spring
poles can be adjacent saplings, branches of a tree, or even poles set
up for that purpose. Refer to the drawing on the following page for
ideas on using spring poles.

I usually tie the snare to my spring pole, and then wrap a piece of
wire to the snare near where it is secured to the pole. This wire is
attached to a notched, wooden peg. When the spring pole is bent
down in place, the peg holds it there by way of a nail driven into a

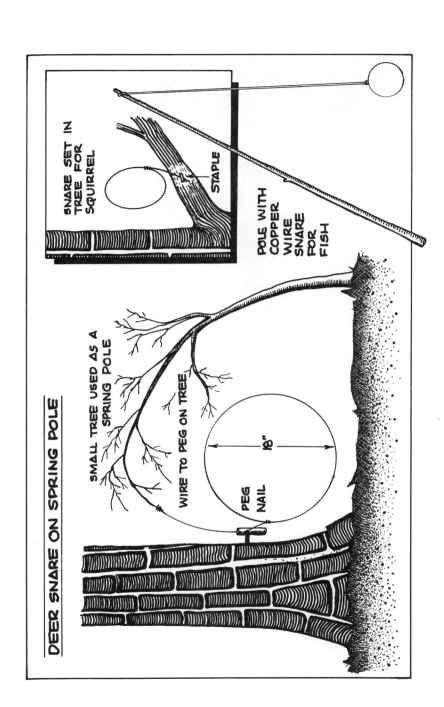

DEER SNARE ON SPRING POLE

SMALL TREE USED AS A SPRING POLE

WIRE TO PEG ON TREE

PEG NAIL

18"

SNARE SET IN TREE FOR SQUIRREL

STAPLE

POLE WITH COPPER WIRE SNARE FOR FISH

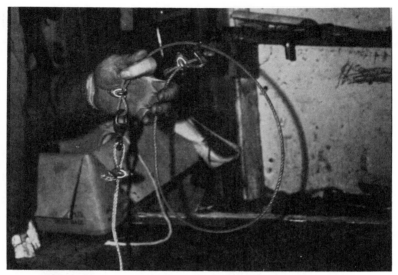

A trapper's bear snare made from steel cable, cable clamps, *L* lock, and a swivel. Ideally, the *L* lock shown should face the opposite direction.

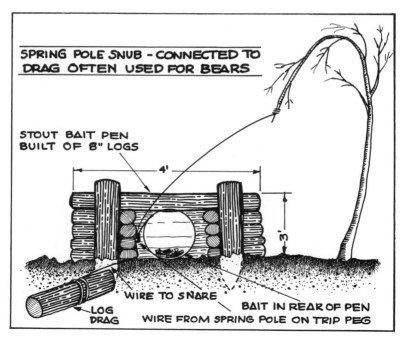

SPRING POLE SNUB - CONNECTED TO DRAG OFTEN USED FOR BEARS

STOUT BAIT PEN BUILT OF 8" LOGS

4'

3'

LOG DRAG

WIRE TO SNARE

BAIT IN REAR OF PEN

WIRE FROM SPRING POLE ON TRIP PEG

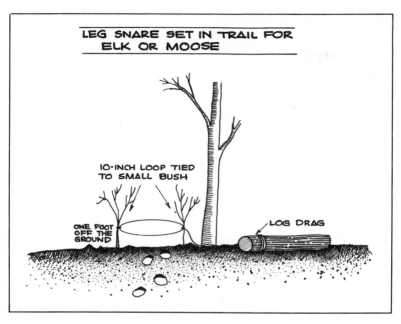

LEG SNARE SET IN TRAIL FOR ELK OR MOOSE

10-INCH LOOP TIED TO SMALL BUSH

ONE FOOT OFF THE GROUND

LOG DRAG

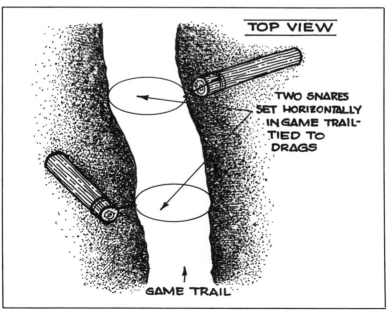

TOP VIEW

TWO SNARES SET HORIZONTALLY IN GAME TRAIL - TIED TO DRAGS

GAME TRAIL

tree or log. The animal then walks into the snare, pulls the peg off the nail, and the pole snaps up and jerks the snare tight.

Larger animals in the moose category are often best taken in snares set horizontally in trails. The catch is made on the leg rather than around the neck. Doing this requires that one set a number of snares close together on regularly used trails. The loop should be much smaller than for deer, about 10 inches in diameter as opposed to about 18 inches for deer. Leg snares are set about 1 foot off the ground. I look for two small bushes about the correct distance apart along the trail. Tie the snare between them with pieces of dead grass.

Instead of a spring pole I just fasten the snare to an 8-inch log about 5 feet long. Not even a bull moose will get very far with a chunk of wood like that dragging along behind him. Sometimes the logs can be used as stepping guides to arrange for the game to put its foot dead into the snare loop.

Bears are often taken in snares. I have seen some very elaborate spring pole snares for bears that attempt to tether the catch till the trapper returns. My advice is not to try and hold any bear in such a stationary setup. They are awfully strong beasts.

Usually I build, or develop if one is naturally available, a small pen that the bear has to go into to get the bait. I set a snare tied to a drag log at the entrance. The only spring pole is a breakaway affair secured with light wire. When the bear hits the snare, the spring pole will trip, snubbing the noose. As soon as the bear fights the loop, it will break the snare away from the spring pole. Then all that holds the bear is the drag log. Drag log marks from bear, elk, and moose are easy to follow through the bush.

Snares are cheap to make and relatively easy to set. Unlike steel traps which must be set very carefully, snares can be virtually strewn around the country. While the catch ratio is low, it doesn't really matter. It's the nature of this survival technology that counts. Set a great number out and you will be guaranteed a few animals.

Deadfalls

One of the light spots in an otherwise dismal world occurs when an environmentalist suggests to me that he intends to head out for the wilderness, and survive by catching game with "Indian deadfalls." I know I won't have to worry about jerks like that competing with me for food the third day after the crash.

Don't get me wrong; deadfalls can indeed be deadly. No question that a family could live on the catch from a line of them. But he who plans to use this kind of trap had better know what the hell he is doing, or said survivalist is going to end up with terminal hunger pangs.

Trigger Designs

The heart of any deadfall is the trigger. My favorite is the figure-four shown in the photograph on page 72. It is a relatively easy-to-make tripping device. More important, it nearly always allows the log to fall unimpeded onto the quarry.

Another good deadfall trigger is the stick and roller. This one must be made of smooth hardwood. The bait stick is fastened above the supporting upright member, which is in place between the drop load and a smooth "roller" on the ground. When the animal pulls the bait, the stick should pop out, throwing the support away from the drop log or rock. Sometimes these triggers have to be set on an angle to make them more sensitive. Experiment with this one.

Triggers of all sorts have been used by trappers. Some are incredibly ingenious. If that's what turns you on, you might experiment with them a bit more. For the average survivor, one more basic design will probably do. It's the trip-stick trigger.

This trigger is used to guard the path of an animal that is passing through. It isn't necessary that the animal grab the bait, just that it hit the trip bar.

Again, the easiest way to learn here is for you to look at the drawings. Be sure to adjust the trip so it goes off with even the slightest pressure. This is much harder than it looks. Rain and snow will change the sensitivity, which can be a big problem with deadfalls.

Deadfall Construction

One of the big problems with deadfalls is the difficulty with constructing very many of them. They last a long time with minimal care, but other than the flat-stone type covered next, take

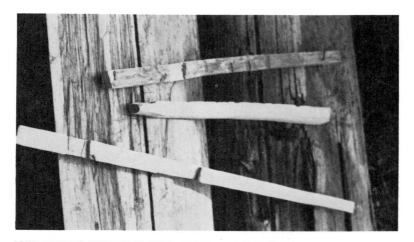

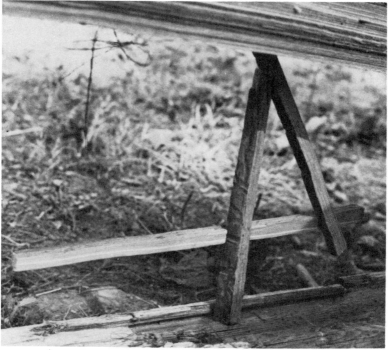

Top: Three sticks needed for figure-four trigger. Note that the longest piece has two notches cut into it.
Bottom: Deadfall with figure-four trigger in place. Bait is wired to the long horizontal piece, which also contains the two notches.

about half a day each to build. This sounds unreasonably long but, in retrospect, it's about what it always takes me.

Also, deadfalls must be set up for a long time before they will produce. Aging improves their kill ratio tremendously. I have built some that never really worked till the third year.

The easiest deadfall to construct and a very good place for the novice to start is by placing figure-four triggers under tilted-up flat rocks. Point the bait stick back under the rock. Add plenty of weight if the existing stone isn't heavy enough.

Whenever I have lived where there are flat rocks that will work for deadfalls, I have gone out in the summer and propped the selected rocks up with plain old sticks. When fall came and I wanted to start collecting game, I substituted the sticks for a figure-four trigger. It's a dynamite way to get possums, skunks, civet cats, weasels, and coons, which are by then accustomed to crawling under the propped-up stones.

Another simple deadfall can be built out of 2-by-8s about 4 feet long. With a trip-stick trigger, it's a pretty good way of guarding a small game run. Just be careful to put the trap in early with as little mess as possible, or the run will be abandoned by the animals.

Use one 2-by-8 for a base plate, and the other for the drop piece. Several guide stakes must be put in on both sides of the deadfall to hold the pieces in line. Heavy rocks must be added to the drop piece to make it lethal.

Conventional deadfalls are made by digging the log base piece at least two-thirds into the ground. The base log can be as short as 4 feet but should be no less than 8 inches in diameter. There has to be something against which to crush the animal. The drop log must be at least 6 to 8 feet long, and no less than 8 inches in diameter. Green, heavy logs are much preferred. Be sure the logs are free from knots and bumps so they fall cleanly.

Usually I construct a rock or log pen behind the trap to protect the bait and steer the animal into the drop zone. Use naturally protective surroundings such as hollow trees, dirt banks, or rock piles if possible.

In snowy climates, it is helpful to cover the trap pen with bark or sticks. One time I had a marten dig down through two feet of snow to get the bait in one of my deadfalls. If I had taken care of

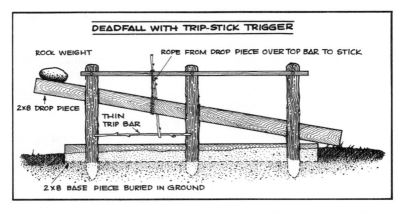

DEADFALL WITH TRIP-STICK TRIGGER

ROCK WEIGHT

ROPE FROM DROP PIECE OVER TOP BAR TO STICK

2x8 DROP PIECE

THIN TRIP BAR

2 X 8 BASE PIECE BURIED IN GROUND

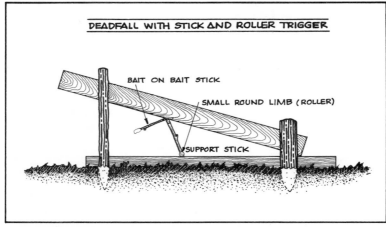

DEADFALL WITH STICK AND ROLLER TRIGGER

BAIT ON BAIT STICK

SMALL ROUND LIMB (ROLLER)

SUPPORT STICK

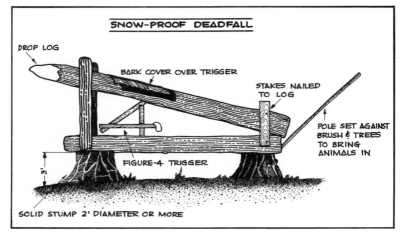

SNOW-PROOF DEADFALL

DROP LOG

BARK COVER OVER TRIGGER

STAKES NAILED TO LOG

POLE SET AGAINST BRUSH & TREES TO BRING ANIMALS IN

3'

FIGURE-4 TRIGGER

SOLID STUMP 2' DIAMETER OR MORE

the trap and kept the snow cleared out, it probably would have wacked it.

Stream Deadfall

At times the survivor can find a place where a tree has fallen in the water across a small stream. To work properly, the log must have sunk in the mud to at least two-thirds of its diameter or more. The tree trunk must be smooth, and yet still be hard to the touch. There won't be many locations with all these criteria. If they are present, though, a very effective stream deadfall can be built.

These sets are quite a bit of work. Before starting, be sure the log is resting on the bottom of the creek all the way across, and that not more than 3 inches of stream water runs over the log. Pound in at least four good stout guide stakes (two per side) and fit with a heavy drop log. Beavers and otters are often bagged in these traps, so lots of weight is required.

Set up a light trip stick a few inches above the water line, and set the trigger. I bend a small sapling down under the drop log with a piece of cloth tied on it. If the flag is up, I know the trap has been sprung, without otherwise going near.

Snow-Proof Deadfall

Old-timers reading this book may remember some of the old deadfall patterns built up on stumps. This style of traps was considered to be snow proof, and in fact is. It works well for marten, squirrels, and coons early in the year. I haven't used the trap much and question whether most survivors will. But for nostalgia's sake, here it is.

Locate two fairly fresh stumps about 10 feet apart. The pair should be at least 2 feet in diameter and level with one another. They should be located not over 15 feet from a fairly dense pine thicket.

Lay an 18-inch base log between the two stumps. Nail 3 stout guide stakes per side, starting from the V-end of the deadfall. The stakes should be 1 foot long near the V, 2 feet in the center, and 3 feet at the end where the log will drop on the animal.

The drop piece should be smaller than the base log. Both members must be free of knots. They have to fall sharply and easily.

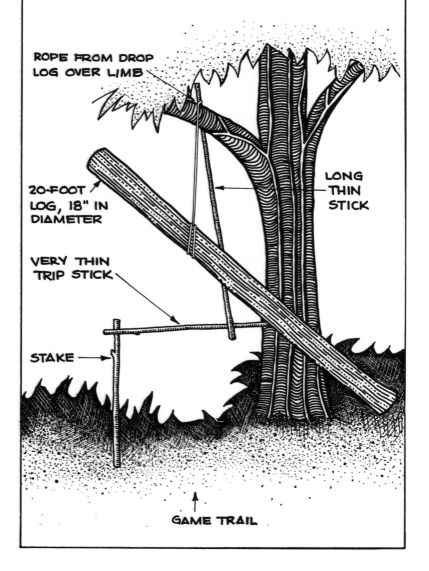

LOG DROP SET IN GAME TRAIL FOR BIG GAME

ROPE FROM DROP
LOG OVER LIMB

LONG
THIN
STICK

20-FOOT
LOG, 18" IN
DIAMETER

VERY THIN
TRIP STICK

STAKE

GAME TRAIL

Set the drop log with a figure-four trigger, with the bait pointed back toward the V under the top log. Cover the trigger-area sides with bark.

Last, find a good limb about 20 feet long. Lean it into the thicket with the butt positioned so the pole touches the stump under the trigger end of the deadfall. This part is important. The critters come much more readily if they can run down out of the trees, along the pole, and enter the trap without going on the ground.

Proper stumps are at least 3 feet high. Theoretically, it will take that much snow to plug the trap. In practice, they will work all winter in snow country.

Survival Log Drop

Those in desperate straits can use a very heavy, long log hoisted up from a stout tree limb to break the backs of deer, elk, or moose. I like snares better, but someday it may be important for you to know about this trap, which is admittedly not a true deadfall. This Log Drop will also smash men, if you need such extra protection around your retreat.

Use a trip-stick trigger with the thinnest crosspiece possible. Set the trap up so the swing stick is at the side of the trail and the trip stick is about 3 feet high. We want the animal to barge through and break the stick rather than push it down.

The only way I have been able to make this trap work consistently is to use a green 18-inch log 20 feet long. Set it up so fully 5 feet of the log hangs out the other side of the path. An ideal setup is from a limb that will allow the log to be hoisted 7 or 8 feet above the path. Four-inch sharpened spikes in the bottom of the log also add effectiveness.

Be sure the kids don't use the path.

Snares and deadfalls are tough traps to use. However, they will work well, and are actually a lot of fun to fool around with. The more traps like these one builds, the more interesting they become.

6. Small Permanent Traps

Smaller animals have good food value, though their calorie content per unit is low. Survivalists who plan to live on smaller game will have to make use of fast, easy collection methods or the effort won't be worth the return.

In some cases the collection techniques outlined in this chapter are desperation measures. They will keep a survivor going when the conditions are initially at their toughest.

Bottle Traps

A good example of a simple little trap that isn't worth a damn except in an emergency situation is the old-fashioned bottle trap. It will catch chipmunks and gophers by the dozens, assuming one is ready to eat these little fellows.

Simply take some one-gallon glass milk jugs with small necks and lay them on their sides wherever chipmunks are. Put four or five whole unshelled peanuts in each bottle for bait.

In short order the chipmunks will start crawling in the bottles trying to get the bait. They will pick up the peanuts and store them in their mouth pouches. A bulging mouth will keep them from getting out of the jar. One can quickly snatch up the jar, trapping them inside.

For years, I have used bottle traps to clear our horse camps of these hungry pests. A camp cook who is on his toes can get rid of all the chipmunks in the area with as few as three or four bottles.

Box Traps

Through the years one of my favorite traps has been the common garden-variety box trap. In my estimation, they are one of the best traps going for the average woodsman. Animals caught in a box trap can be released unharmed if that is appropriate. At other times

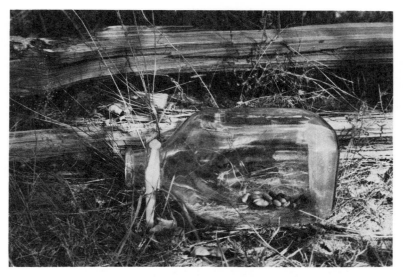

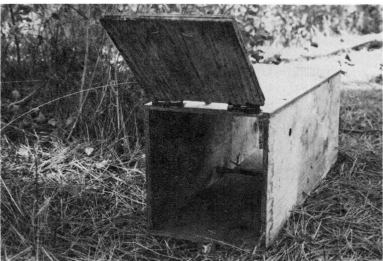

Top: Milk jug trap for chipmunks and ground squirrels. Bait is peanuts or other nuts.

Bottom: A simple homemade box trap. Note trip bar in center of box's interior. A string running upward from the trip bar holds up both end doors until animal touches bait on trip bar. Doors are then released, trapping the quarry.

it might be wise to place the catch in holding pens for fattening and subsequent slaughter. Sometimes this is possible with steel traps, but I wouldn't count on it.

Wooden, home-built box traps are cheap. We make ours from whatever material is lying around. Once built, modestly maintained and protected, they last for years.

Other animals can't get at the catch in a box trap. I shudder to think of how many times I have had magpies ruin a mink, marten, or weasel in a steel trap. When the predatory animals are of the two-legged variety, box traps that hide the catch are especially important. Today few people have any idea what in the world the little wooden contraptions are.

The best box traps have open ends. Critters can see through end to end and will be less fearful about coming in. In this regard, box traps appeal to many animals. Placed next to buildings, in brush heaps, board piles, along fence rows, under overhanging banks and creeks, the box can appear to be a sheltered run. Small animals like the idea of moving through protected places similar to the inside of a box trap. At times I have felt they were taking refuge in the trap when they were caught.

Transportation is the biggest problem with box traps. It's tough to carry them around to all the places where a trap could be set. Three or four are good to have set around one's home or retreat. Thirty or forty on a normal trap line are ridiculous to transport and maintain. Things would have to be pretty grim before I would start thinking about stringing that many out across the countryside.

Skunks, rabbits, squirrels, possums, and woodchucks are fairly easy to catch in a box trap. Coyotes, fox, beavers, and the exotics (marten, fisher, otter, and badger) are pretty much impossible. Coons, muskrats, and mink fall in the middle. I would guess that most seasoned trappers would think mink are virtually impossible to catch in a homemade trap. Through the years I have picked up a mink now and then, attributable in most cases to the care with which I handle my boxes, and to the sensitivity I build into the trigger.

Box traps should be constructed ahead of the time of use, and then set out in the rain and snow to age. When moving them, don't put the trap under your arm or over your shoulder. Wear gloves

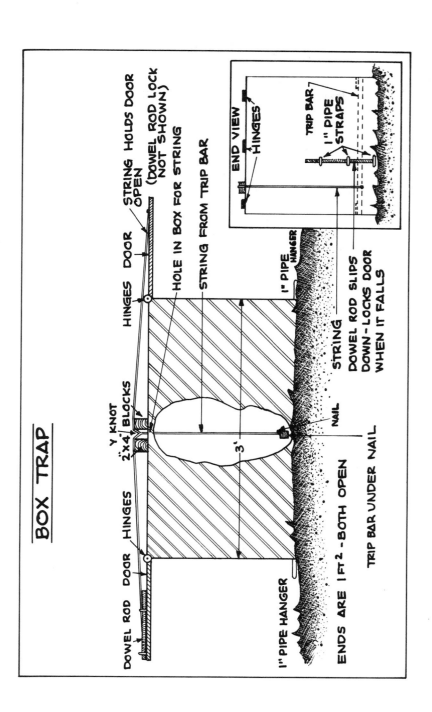

BOX TRAP

DOWEL ROD DOOR HINGES

Y KNOT
2"x 4" BLOCKS

HINGES DOOR

STRING HOLDS DOOR OPEN

(DOWEL ROD LOCK NOT SHOWN)

HOLE IN BOX FOR STRING

STRING FROM TRIP BAR

1" PIPE HANGER

STRING

DOWEL ROD SLIPS DOWN — LOCKS DOOR WHEN IT FALLS

NAIL

3'

1" PIPE HANGER

ENDS ARE 1 FT² — BOTH OPEN

TRIP BAR UNDER NAIL

END VIEW

HINGES

TRIP BAR

1" PIPE STRAPS

and use a temporary wire handle. Just avoid touching the trap as much as possible. After the trap is set, leave it in place at least two months. This means you will have to set it in the correct area the first time.

The traps that work best for me are the ones with an opening about 10 inches square. Many times the availability of scrap materials dictates the size here more than anything else, so giving an approximate size is always judicious. Length is also very important. To work well, the trap should be either very short, or very long. Some single-door traps with wire backs are good performers. Two-door traps are best constructed in the 4-foot-long range. Use good sound wood. Some animals can chew like mini-chain saws. They can reduce rotten pine to shavings in a matter of hours.

Always use two hinges on each door, or the catch will squirm through the sides and escape.

Skunks caught in box traps can safely be carried to a convenient pool of water and drowned. It's the only gauranteed scentless method of dispatching these creatures that I know of.

Sometimes I use bait in the traps. Other times, if the set is placed in a run or along an old barn, I don't.

Muskrats are at times attracted to fresh sweet corn, carrots, or dried corn. Coons like sardines or peanut butter. Mink will come in to a live mouse. I can't get rabbits to come to any kind of bait. They just seem to wander in when they darn well please. Buckeyes or acorns are great for squirrels. Woodchucks like carrots, and possums like apples or peanut butter, and so on. Generally try to figure out what the quarry in your area eat and serve them that.

Raccoon Spike Trap

The raccoon spike trap is another inexpensive yet effective trap that can be made with cheap, easily obtainable materials.

Originally my uncle showed me how to make these traps in a small version. They worked modestly well for coons. Later when I was older, I got to follow him around his line of bear spike traps. It came as quite a shock to discover his bear traps were essentially the same as the coon version but, of course, much larger.

Tools required are a hand auger with a 1-inch bit, a file, hammer, and some nails. Uncle used to make his coon traps in fallen logs or in solid stumps and roots. Until I saw the bear traps, I never realized they could be portable.

The design, like everything good in life, is simplicity itself. Start by drilling a 1-inch diameter hole in a solid block of wood (8-inch section of 4-by-4 is ideal), or the solid log or stump you have decided on for a natural location. Blocks have the advantage of being portable, but are much harder to catch coons in unless they are large. If the hole is sunk into a log or stump, put it in vertically or at least tipped up vertically. I don't think a horizontal hole will work. Drill the hole in at least 6 inches deep. Portable spike trap blocks that a coon could carry away must be wired down to a stake or drag log.

Sharpen four 12-penny nails to needlepoints and drive them into and around the hole till the points come within 3/8-inch of touching. The nails should reach this point about 2½ inches down in the augered hole. Adjustments can be made by bending the nails a bit after they are driven in. Hair, stolen bait, or other evidence of a missed coon should prompt one to further adjust the trap.

Bait with quail blood or honey. Be sure the bait falls all the way down to the bottom of the hole.

One hundred of these spike traps is not an unreasonable number. That many will catch 60 percent of the coons within three miles of your retreat. You will also catch a few oppossums and an occasional skunk.

Turtle Trap

Survivalists who are familiar with standard freshwater fish traps will recognize a turtle trap immediately. Turtle traps are much the same except for the funnel opening, mesh size, and depth.

Nylon net versions are available commercially. Cost is about twenty-five dollars. In my estimation, the nylon types are inferior when actually used for turtles rather than fish. Big old snappers make mincemeat out of them.

I suggest making your own from ⅜-inch rebar bent into 3-foot hoops, and covered with 2-inch fur farm wire. If this heavier grade of chicken wire isn't available, use standard welded wire.

Bait the turtle trap with anything rotten, such as dead cats, fish heads, or squirrel guts.

8484844

84844844

84444

44

444

84 the drawing that this trap is large—7 or 8 feet long. It has two funnels separated by a 2-foot gap. Turtles are notorious trap busters, but they don't get out of this one. I have even left a couple of large leatherbacks in a trap like the one shown for a couple of weeks. They stored well till I had a chance to make a big pot of turtle stew with them.

Prawn Trap

I have used this trap in rocky reefs and coral beds from eastern Florida around to the Gulf and from California up to northern British Columbia. It is much like a fish or turtle trap yet different enough to really do a good job on prawns (shrimp). For some reason the solid boards on two sides create a situation that the shrimp like a lot more than a plain old wire trap.

Start with two 18-by-14-inch pieces of ⅝-inch marine plywood. Nail or screw securely together, so the resulting piece forms an L. Cover the open length of the L with ½-inch hardware screen. Fasten one end piece on with wire. Make it removable, since this is where the captured prawns are removed. The cone which goes into the opposite end must be very long and slender. It should reach at least 3 feet into the trap. End diameter is about 3 inches. Finish the prawn trap by wrapping two pieces of number 9 wire around it to use as a handle.

Rocks or metal must be used to sink the box. I get the best results in 80 to 100 feet of water. Bait the trap with a chopped cod or other fish bait. On several occasions I have even caught octopuses in these rigs.

Fridge Trap

An unusual trap that is surprisingly effective can be built using an old refrigerator. I have caught numerous coons in my fridge trap located in a dump near my present home. All I did was lay the refrigerator on its back and prop the door open with a figure-four trigger. Bait is a piece of sardine or peanut butter. About half the time the trigger pieces don't clear. They keep the door from latching, allowing the coon to escape. Under the circumstances, I don't view that as much of a problem. It didn't take me five minutes to set this outfit up. The coons always seem to be back the next night.

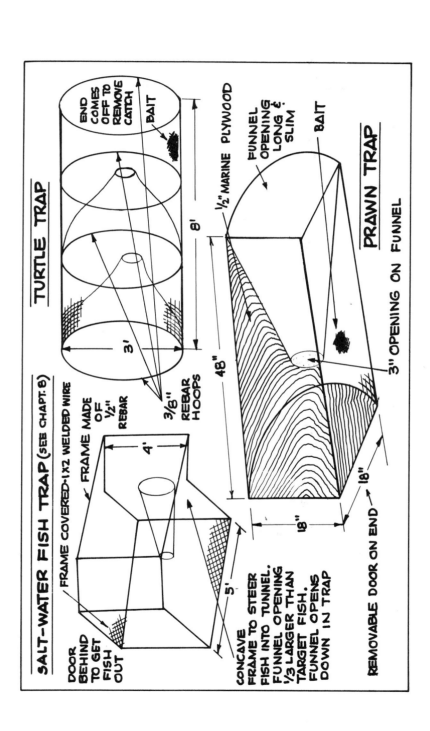

SALT-WATER FISH TRAP (SEE CHAPT. 8)

TURTLE TRAP

FRAME COVERED-1x2 WELDED WIRE

DOOR BEHIND TO GET FISH OUT

FRAME MADE OF

4'

5'

CONCAVE FRAME TO STEER FISH INTO TUNNEL. FUNNEL OPENING ⅓ LARGER THAN TARGET FISH. FUNNEL OPENS DOWN IN TRAP

END COMES OFF TO REMOVE CATCH

BAIT

8'

3'

FRAME MADE OF ½" REBAR

⅜" REBAR HOOPS

48"

½" MARINE PLYWOOD

FUNNEL OPENING LONG & SLIM

BAIT

3" OPENING ON FUNNEL

PRAWN TRAP

18"

18"

REMOVABLE DOOR ON END

Tree Dens and Hollow Logs

Not too far from where I live now, there is a hollow log. Actually, there are a number of hollow logs around the woods near here. My particular hollow log, however, is different.

Every time I have looked inside, a nice fat rabbit has been waiting for me. Usually I have been able to convert the rabbit to rabbit stew in short order.

Originally my Airedale found the log while chasing a rabbit. I obliged him and ran the hare out, giving the hound a chance to resume the race. Next time we were in the area I made a point of looking in the log; sure enough, more food. While hollow logs and den trees are not traps themselves, they are very nearly one if treated properly. The trick is to find the den trees and logs that are frequented by game. Not all hollow logs attract game. Old-time coon and squirrel hunters don't have to be told how to find den trees. If you know some of these people, don't read the next few paragraphs. Go ask one of these experts.

Good den-tree finders look for tracks in the mud and snow, beaten down paths, chips of bark at the bases of trees, freshly chipped tree trunks and, naturally, the dens themselves. Sometimes one can even find a few pieces of hair on the log or tree. Certain trees characteristically are more likely to have dens in them, but don't always count on it.

Hollow logs that attract game are usually characterized by odd, obscured entrances. The log den I mentioned is in a large curved oak branch perhaps 14 inches in diameter. One of the curved ends is open, but points down toward the ground. The large limb makes a little loop where another branch broke off years before, and rotted out, thus forming a perfect hiding place for rabbits. They run under the log and crawl up into the hollow from underneath. This bottom entrance makes it especially attractive to game that is trying to hide.

Most dens are too high up in the trees to reach without special climbing equipment. However, by persistently looking hard and using the services of my faithful pooch, I always seem to be able to locate a couple of good dens in my territory that are relatively easy to reach. One notable example is in a giant old willow tree. It has large, steplike branches that lead up 20 feet to the den opening. The opening is about 8 inches in diameter and 3 feet deep. Another is in a giant walnut up about 8 feet off the ground. We simply put a log against the tree to climb up for a look.

Some dens are used constantly. No matter how many times I move or where I live, two or three like this always turn up. Right now we have a dandy coyote den located in a draw not two miles from where I live. I have been able to call two or three of the varmints out every year.

Ground dens that are being used will have beaten paths up to them. There will be fresh digging, hair, some smell, worn edges, and droppings.

Once the active dens, hollow trees, and logs in the area are spotted, it is simple to make the harvest with a club or .22. Again, to make this work, you must *know the territory*.

7. Using Steel Traps

Probably many of the people who read this book won't need a simple primer on steel traps which snap shut on an animal's leg. I, for one, take them so much for granted that I don't even have extra traps stashed with my survival gear or in my caches. We have enough around that I can't imagine not being able to come up with six or eight any time I need them. Also, leg-hold traps are almost universally available from dozens of sources.

Steel traps are important to the survivor, but I often question just how important they are. They *are* handy, and require less skill than a snare to use. On the other hand, steel traps are relatively expensive, complex enough to foul up with maddening frequency, and of a nature that immediately makes many animals suspicious.

I do know of one steel trap set that my old uncle taught me which I have never seen in print. It's a dynamite trick for hard-to-catch animals like coyote, mink, and fox. As a bonus to those who stick with me during my simple little explanation of steel traps, I have described this set at the end of the chapter.

The concept of the standard steel trap has been around for hundreds of years. I have seen some traps in Turkey that the sultans used, made in the 1500s. Tempering the spring steel was always the problem that kept these early iron traps from working dependably. Often these crude traps would shatter when sprung in cold water, or on frozen ground. At the very best, they lost their power after being set but a short time.

About 1820 a small commune of religious folks near Oneida, New York, developed and marketed a steel trap with a tempered spring that could withstand months of being set in cold, inhospitable conditions. The steel traps we have today are descendents of those Oneida traps. In most respects, the design is identical.

Steel Trap Types

Basically there are three types of steel traps that catch the critter by the foot. They are the long-spring trap, the coil-spring trap, and the jump trap.

Most common is the long-spring trap. They, as the name implies, have a long, flat spring that closes the jaws of the trap. Small ones have a small spring, medium ones a little bigger spring, and so on. After size number 2 the traps are built with two springs, and are appropriately called double long-spring traps.

Sizes of these traps run from the little "0" used for rats and weasels, through to a number 4 double spring that will hold large beaver and wolves. I have even caught a small bear in a number 4 double long-spring.

Before 1940, the various trap companies made large 12- to 35-pound long-spring bear traps. I have a few around that are now sought-after antiques; they are too valuable to put out in the bush. Besides, there are better, easier ways of catching bears than in these monstrous steel contraptions.

The other side of the coin—and a steel trap that I don't recommend—is the coil spring. These traps derive their holding power from coil springs rather than from flat springs. Often the coils will weaken and break after only limited use, especially if the trap is used in water sets.

It is my understanding that coil-spring traps were first developed for fox. They are a good bet in dens or anyplace where space is limited, if you can easily go to the store and buy new ones when the old ones wear out.

Manufacture of coil-spring traps seems irregular. A few years back I saw a quantity of number 3s offered for sale. Before that time I had never seen a coil spring in any size except a 1½ or a 2. Since then, some 1s have turned up and the 3s have become common. It is hard for me to tell what the average reader may run into as far as coil-spring traps go.

The third type of trap is the jump, or under-spring, model. On the whole, these are pretty good game-getters. They take less space and are easier to set than long springs. Here the problem is the relative speed with which their springs lose power. It is not as great as with coil springs, but is still a negative factor, especially when set in water.

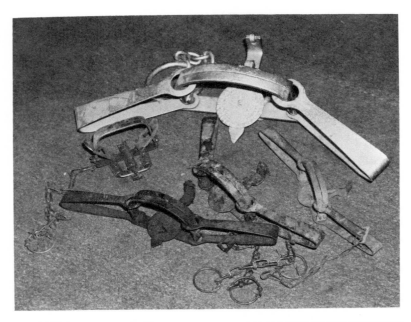

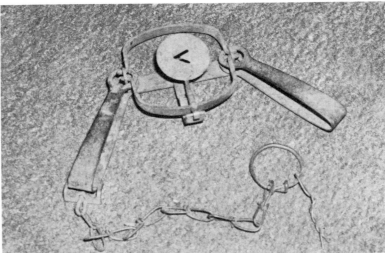

Top: A giant antique bear trap dwarfs two number 4 coyote traps in the foreground, a number 2 coil-spring trap on the left, and an old number 2 double long-spring on the right.
Bottom: A number 4 double long-spring steel trap set and ready to go.

Jump traps are made in all sizes from 0 up to number 4s. When I was in my mid-teens I finally saved enough money to buy a number 3 jump, which was my big gun reserved for special occasions.

Through the years I had a lot of fun with that trap. I caught a number of badgers, as well as a coyote or two and an otter. I still had the trap the year I was thirty, when we were forced to auction off our farm and equipment. It broke something inside me when the auctioneer put my faithful old trap on the block and sold it off. Everything went but the clothes on our backs, but I most vividly remember that old trap going.

Killer Traps

Around the turn of the century there were a number of manufacturers who sold killer traps, rather than leg-hold models. Gradually they dropped this type of trap. By the 1920s, killer traps were considered antiques. Then about twenty years ago, the conibear traps hit the market and we were back in the killer-trap business again.

Probably because I am an old duffer, set in my ways, I don't much like conibear traps, other than in special limited applications. They are difficult to set properly and, in my opinion, fairly dangerous. Lest you think this is a blanket condemnation, let me add that I have a few conibear traps and know a few trappers who use them.

Trap Selection

Would-be trappers should try to get by with as few different sizes as possible. I use number 1½ long-springs for muskrats, coons, skunks, possums, weasels, civet cats, groundhogs, nutrias, turtles, squirrels, cats, and mink.

Coyotes, fox, beaver, and bobcats can be caught just fine in number 2 traps. By keeping my trap inventory down to two sizes I can change parts and cannibalize old traps easily. I'll have something to trap with long after the guy who has one or two of everything.

Steel Trap Care and Maintenance

To keep them in top shape, steel traps should be boiled and waxed. This process prevents them from rusting, adds lubrication, and kills the human scent on them. I boil all my traps once a year.

Put the traps in a container that can safely be boiled for two days. Cover with water and add about 5 cups of walnut hulls or native tree bark per 10 gallons of water. Boil slowly for two days, or until the traps take on a blue-black hue.

At the end of the boiling cycle, throw in 1 pound of paraffin and half a pound of beeswax for every 100 traps. Use a wire to pull the traps out of the boiling mixture through the boiling liquid. The hot wax will flow onto the traps, providing a thin, tough coating that is difficult to detect.

Treated traps should be hung in a barn or under a tree, away from contact with humans, to minimize scent problems later on.

Setting Steel Traps

Never, under any condition, set any steel trap smaller than a number 3 by stepping on the spring. Depress the spring with your hands and flop the jaws over to hold it. Standing on a trap will decrease its life considerably.

After latching the *dog* to the *pan* on a long-spring trap, twist the spring toward the pan. This flattens the trap out and makes a better, neater package. The trap must now be attached to something to prevent the game from running off with it.

Since some of these traps are either a bit small or a bit large, I like to attach my trap to a drag log rather than staking it down permanently. Drags are not as visible as stakes, often protecting the trap and game from thieves. Land animals such as coyotes or bobcats will pull a drag into the bush and wait quietly, thinking they are hidden.

Some of the traps I use are large enough to break the animal's leg. Muskrats, for instance, will chew their front leg off and get away under those circumstances if the trap is staked down. With the trap attached to a floating stick or small log, however, the rat will swim out in deep water and drown before that happens. Beaver can pull out of a number 2 trap. But with the trap wired to a floating log that just drifts around the pond, the beaver won't be able to break loose.

In the Field

There are essentially two types of steel trap sets in the field: bait sets that attract the animals into the trap, and run sets that take

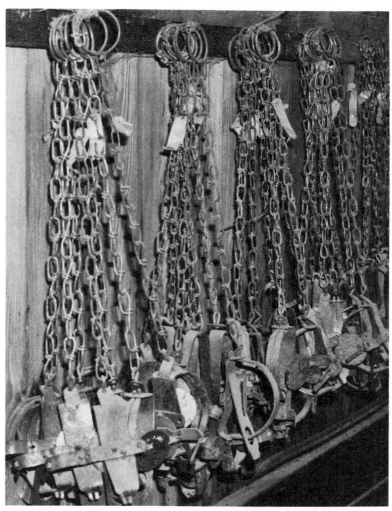

A workshop wall lined with dozens of steel traps, ranging in size from number 1s to number 4s. These traps can help provide the survivalist and his family with food, clothing, and other outdoor products. Steel traps are also good trading stock, since they cannot be made without special metal-forming and heat-treating equipment. They are therefore choice items to be cached away against the day of need.

advantage of the fact that the game uses a regular path. Both types of sets require a good, in-depth knowledge of the animal, its eating habits, and how it lives.

A good place to start is with muskrats, which are abundant. They are also easy to trap and good to eat. Mostly muskrats are caught in run sets. I suggest the novice trapper who knows he will have to survive by trapping start practicing on these animals.

Woodchucks are easy to trap in dens during the summer. Coons, skunks, and possums come to bait quite readily. Continue your land set practice on these mammals.

Remember to always cover the trap. Leave as little scent and disturbance as possible, and trap where you know there are animals to be caught.

I should add here that this is not intended to be a text on trapping. Good, comprehensive books on trapping are available at your library. I strongly urge you to read some of them and then get out and practice.

Uncle's Secret Set

Now for my uncle's secret steel trap set. Experts, please bear with me. I will go into a great deal of detail for the benefit of the novice who may never have set a trap before in his life.

The set is called a *live-mouse set*. It is a dandy for coyote, fox, badger, coon, bobcat, mink, possum, and skunks. I honestly know of no better set that has ever been developed for all of these creatures.

The most difficult part of the project can be catching the required live mouse. Survivors are probably going to have lots of mice around. If you make it that far, I don't think the live mouse is going to be an insurmountable problem.

Gently place the live mouse in a large fruit or mayonnaise jar that has previously been well cleaned. Punch holes in the lid, and pour in at least one handful of grain and two or three of dry grass. Make the jar as homey as possible for the mouse. Next wrap a piece of cloth around the jar so the mouse won't be frightened and die. Don't shake or jolt the jar after the mouse is in it.

Tie a double 4-foot piece of number 16 wire to the chain ring of a number 2 long-spring trap. Now set this arrangement aside.

MOUSE IN BOTTLE SET

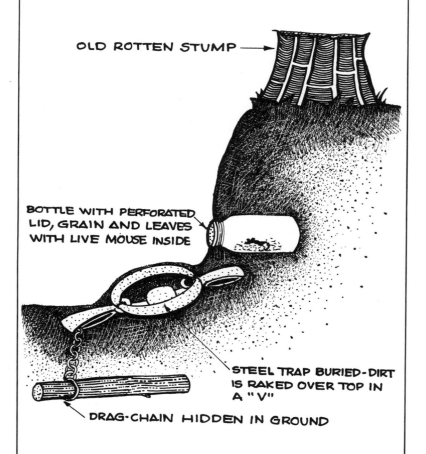

OLD ROTTEN STUMP →

BOTTLE WITH PERFORATED LID, GRAIN AND LEAVES WITH LIVE MOUSE INSIDE

STEEL TRAP BURIED-DIRT IS RAKED OVER TOP IN A "V"

DRAG-CHAIN HIDDEN IN GROUND

Dig a small, horizontal hole back into a dry sheltered bank under a rotted stump or other similar sheltered dry place, where a mouse den might occur naturally. Tip the jar onto its long side and put it in the hole, burying all but the perforated cap.

All extra dirt must be piled on a piece of burlap or deer hide on which the trapper himself kneels to prepare the set. Don't ever touch the ground with your hands, smoke, or spit. Digging can be done with a small trowel or with a hand ax.

Hollow out an area 8 inches in front of the mouse bottle just deep enough to hold the steel trap. Place the trap in the hold, and cover it with a big leaf and then lightly with dirt and duff. Rake some loose dirt from the mouse hole in a V over the trap so it looks like some other animal dug there.

Cut a small channel for the trap chain and wire. These must be buried in the channel out of sight. Double-wire the chain onto a 3-inch log 4 feet long. This drag should be placed back from the set in a natural-looking way.

The set will last till the mouse has been dead a week. Sometimes this can be as long as five weeks or more. Uncle's secret set is deadly on big old ridge-running mink, or coyotes that are normally very difficult to trap.

Like most good sets, this one is fairly simple. It should be checked every other day, but always from afar. Don't go tramping by the set leaving tracks, scent, and debris, and then wonder why nothing ever comes in and gets caught.

Freezing ground or blowing snow sometimes will make this set inoperative. I try to locate mouse sets in sheltered areas where I can enclose the trap with rotten dry wood to minimize the problem.

Steel Traps—A Final Note

Skillful use of steel traps is going to be very important to some survivors. If all of this is new to you, I strongly urge that you purchase a few additional books on trapping. Start in now and learn. Catching a muskrat isn't much of a trick after you have once done it. Getting up in the morning after the collapse with the intention of going trapping for dinner is unrealistic to the extreme, without proper preparations.

8. Emergency Fish and Fowl

In a desperate survival situation, with no caches to fall back on, I would look first to the fishes and then to the birds for food to tide me over till I could get my total program rolling. Almost every pond, slough, lake, and stream in North America is home for some kind of fish. They may not be game fish, but after missing three or four meals in a row I would have no qualms at all about throwing a bucket of three-inch bluegills, or bullheads, in a pot and making fish stew.

There are several practical ways to proceed if one needs to collect fish in a hurry. The suggestions below are in rough order of inverse complexity. Those that require the least preparation and equipment are listed first.

Fish "Hogging"

How many people reading this book are familiar with the terms "hogging," or "feeling" for fish? Some of the real old-timers may remember that this was considered to be a reasonably good way of catching catfish, suckers, gar, and carp—all plentiful species.

The procedure is simple enough. One wades the large creeks and small rivers looking for submerged hollow logs and cutouts under the banks—anyplace where fish might hide. Work upstream and watch out for water snakes. Try as much as possible to stay in four feet or less of water. This is not a diving method.

When a likely place is found, carefully squat down in the water and feel around with your hands. If the smooth, plastic-textured surface of a fish is felt, proceed very gently. Be cautious not to poke the fish with a finger. Touching does not seem to scare them, but jabbing will.

Having located the fish, there are three ways to go. You can try slipping a copper wire snare on the fish's tail, getting a finger in a gill, or a hand in the mouth. Use a thin leather glove if it's catfish or gar. These fish can really tear up a person's hands.

This method works surprisingly well in the summer when getting wet isn't a problem, and the fish are hot and sluggish. It is, on the other hand, an art and takes practice to perfect.

A similar technique—feeling under stream banks for turtles—is useful in some areas. It is also dangerous if water moccasins inhabit the area. One simply works along the banks feeling up underneath for the mossy, hard shells of turtles. If you find one, work your fingers over the top of the shell. Quickly grasp the shell at the top end and pull it out. Remember that a big snapper can take off the end of a finger like it was a hotdog; this method has its disadvantages.

Rock Trap

Rock traps that funnel fish into pen-barriers, built across creeks and small rivers, work well. Building one of these traps requires a lot of labor, but has the distinct advantage of being semi-permanent without requiring special tools or materials. See the facing illustration for construction details.

Sometimes rock traps can be built in a bay or in a small stream that connects two larger bodies of water. I built one between two lakes about fifteen miles from Eagle River, Wisconsin, some thirty years ago. Part of the trap was a beaver dam. Two of the V's were nothing more than a series of heavy stakes driven into the soft mud. The final barrier was a wall of stone. I got some bass, a few trout, and a bunch of pike in the trap over the course of one summer.

Excellent rock traps can be built in natural estuaries, river mouths, and bays along the coast. In my estimation, they can provide a very good, easy way of collecting fish from the ocean. The only real problem is finding the correct set of natural conditions in which to build the trap. Rock traps require too much labor to be put in any old place indiscriminately.

Fish Spears

Survivalists who don't have one should either make or buy a good fish spear. Be selective when you acquire a spear. There should be four or five fairly heavy tines, at least 5 inches long. The entire spear should weigh about 2 pounds and be 5 to 6 inches wide.

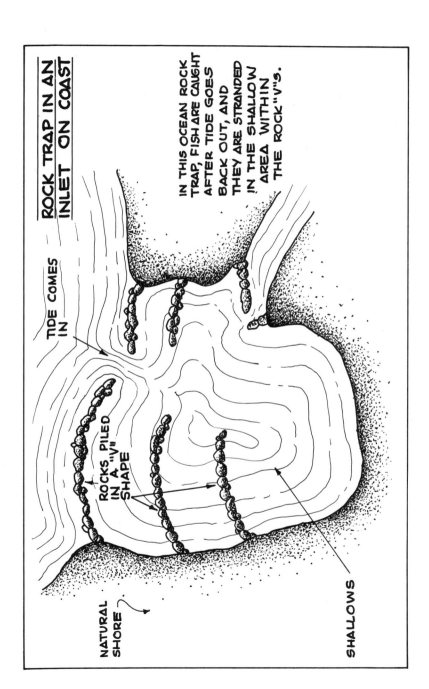

ROCK TRAP IN AN INLET ON COAST

IN THIS OCEAN ROCK TRAP, FISH ARE CAUGHT AFTER TIDE GOES BACK OUT, AND THEY ARE STRANDED IN THE SHALLOW AREA WITHIN THE ROCK "V"S.

TIDE COMES IN

ROCKS PILED IN A "V" SHAPE

NATURAL SHORE

SHALLOWS

Provision should be made to attach a stout 6-foot removable handle.

In conjunction with a fish spear I sometimes use the techniques of hanging a light over the water to attract fish. Another less known wrinkle is to hang the light down *in* the water. This approach works especially well in the ocean. I use a waterproof aluminum 6-cell police flashlight, tied to a piece of ⅜-inch nylon rope. A few years back my son-in-law was experimenting with this method and lost a fifty-dollar flashlight with rechargeable batteries to a big hungry mouth. The 25-pound fish line he was using didn't stop the lunker—whatever it was—for an instant.

Try hanging the light in about 3 feet of water and spearing whatever comes in. If that doesn't work, lower the light to about 20 feet and work it up gradually. This either works well or not at all, depending on the fish in the area.

Shooting Fish

Sometimes fish can be shot with a rifle. This is a tricky business requiring a fair degree of skill. It can also waste a lot of ammo in a hurry. Some bullets won't penetrate the water very well, which in turn distorts the fish's whereabouts. Remember that fish in the water are closer and lower than they appear to be. One must aim under the image to get a hit.

Larger, heavier bullets, thrown at modest velocities, work best. I like to use a .38 Special rifle one of my boys has to shoot carp. We load it with a reduced powder charge and heavy gas-checked bullets.

Sometimes a bow and fish arrow can be used to collect a meal. It's about the only realistic survival use of a bow I know of.

Trot Lines

Trot (or set) lines work well in some circumstances for fish. A trot line is nothing more than a heavy piece of line strung with a number of smaller side lines attached to baited hooks. Some trot lines in large lakes may have as many as two thousand hooks.

Bait and hook size must be applicable to the fish one is trying to catch. Baiting number 2 hooks with liver and corn is a good general compromise. Be sure you know what fish the water you have in mind supports, so you can put the trot line in where the fish are likely to be. Ths is part of your presurvival inventory that you should be doing now. Check the line every few days, and rebait as needed.

Fish Trap

Fish traps, once they are built, provide lots of calories with a minimum of effort. The ocean fish trap (page 85) is much larger than needed for most freshwater fish. Something similar but smaller (page 102) should be built for inland lakes and streams.

I build my fish trap frames out of ½-inch steel rebar of the type used for concrete reinforcements. The wire covering should be no more than 1-by-2-inch mesh for use in the ocean. This is a standard welded-wire size. Freshwater coverings are ideally made from ½-inch chicken wire.

Be sure the funnel side of the ocean fish trap is concave. This is important so that the fish are steered toward the entrance.

The outer perimeter of the entrance funnel should be about a third larger in diameter than the size of fish you hope to catch. Inside, the funnel narrows to approximately the size of the fish. The opening must point down level with the floor of the trap. Be sure to put in an easy-access door, to get the catch out.

I like to set these traps in about 20 feet of water and check them by diving, rather than hauling them out. Off the Mexican coast, we had one trap about 10 feet by 5 feet, and 4 feet deep, that bagged dozens of pounds of fish a day while we kept it going.

Bait the fish trap with hog liver, deer entrails, other fish guts, or anything bloody. In fresh water I use an old squirrel carcass, fish heads, or even an ear of fresh corn.

Nets and Netting

Nets are valuable survival tools. If they are on hand, caching a good supply of food can be easy. Later in this chapter I will give a basic set of instructions on how to make a net. Because the process requires a special set of materials and an inordinate amount of time, it isn't always too practical. Yet readers should at least have a working knowledge of nets so they can repair them, if nothing else.

It is better by far to cache nets now rather than trying to scrounge materials later. If your territory is such that nets of one kind or another will be needed, buy and store them now.

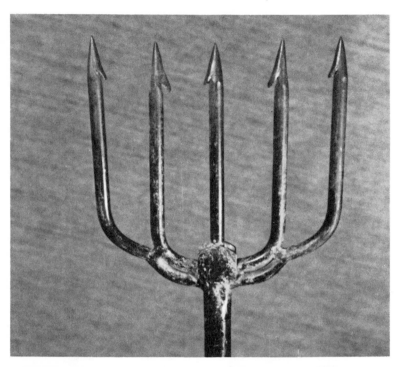

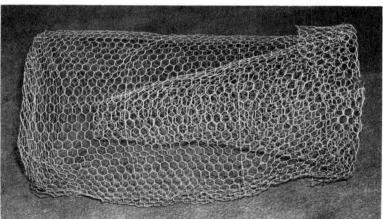

Top: Heavy-duty fish spear ordered from outdoor supply house. The tines are five inches high, and spaced an inch-and-a-half apart. Total weight of the spearhead is one pound.
Bottom: Freshwater fish trap made from ½-inch chicken wire, hog rings, and number 9 wire.

Dip seines are the easiest net to make and use. They can be nothing more than a 6-foot piece of ½-inch chicken wire, a drapery, bedspread, or even a sheet tied up with four lines to a pole.

Bait and a few rocks are placed in the center of the seine. The rig is lowered slowly to the bottom. Pull the rig when you see a fish cross, or every five minutes or so. If no fish are taken, change territory, bait, or method.

Gill nets are devices that trap the fish around the gills when they try to swim through the net webbing. There is a fairly severe sorting for size, since the little fish pass through and the bigger ones are turned back by the barrier.

Floats are secured to the top of the gill net to hold it up. Lead weights secured on the bottom keep it from buckling and billowing in the water. At times gill nets are used without weights. They are set across rivers or in bays on rigid lines (generally steel cable) at a predetermined depth. The lines are set so the net is held taut at the proper depth.

Several firms are now making small trawl nets. These nets take long hours to make at home. If you think you will have a power boat to use, there is nothing better for catching lots of fish. In most cases so many fish will be caught in a very short time that you will want to either be in a co-op with other families, or you should be prepared to trade fish for something. Of course, if there is no fuel to run your boat, you are out of luck.

It takes about 1.5 horsepower per foot of net width at the net's mouth to pull a trawl. A small 10-foot trawl net can be pulled for a short time by four stout rowers. If there are plenty of fish around, this muscle-powered method will work. It never really works well, however. Under some circumstances I understand a trawl can be pulled by a boat under sail. It's worth looking into.

Freshwater trawls work great pulled along the edge of weed beds early in spring for pike, or in deep water for perch and walleye. If the bottom is clear, they will catch bass. At the mouths of rivers, they will even pick up trout, salmon, and dolly varden. Along the coast a trawl is the best thing I know of for fish like rays, whiting, and catfish that live in the shallow surfy water. The only prerequisite for operating a small trawl net is that the ocean bottom be fairly obstacle-free.

Trawls can be made out of nursery netting, chicken wire, mesh cloth, or anything else that the ingenious survivor can come up with. Right now they are not expensive to purchase. If a trawl would fit into your survival package, you might consider going the commercial route. They *are* time consuming to make from scratch. Sea Isle Net Company (129 Druid Oaks Lane, Box 570, St. Simons Island, GA, 31522) sells a full line of quality trawl nets. Those who have to knit their own trawls should refer to the drawing. A trawl works best in about 25 feet of water. I have, at times, run mine down to 75 feet. The rule of thumb is to use 3 feet of towline for every foot of desired depth.

Gill nets and trawls are fairly sophisticated in concept. Many survivalists may not have even thought of using them. Even a dip seine is a bit bewildering the first time out. There are many other nets that do a fine job that won't be covered in this book. Food foragers who know they will need nets might be advised to spend some additional time researching the subject in the library.

The last net I will cover is the good old, simple, everyday seine. These nets are simply barriers that are pulled or pushed through the water in a manner that will enclose or trap fish. Little 8-foot models for use on minnows and other bait in small streams can be made out of two sticks, two pieces of rope, and some loose-weave drapery cloth. Weights aren't even required.

The sticks are tied on the ends of the rope. Whatever comprises the net is tied between the top and bottom ropes. Two men push the sticks upstream through the water, keeping the net taut. Larger rocks in the net's path are passed over. That's all there is to it.

Larger nets have floats on top, weights on the bottom, plywood side doors, and rope ends to pull on with no side sticks. These longer seines can be used to drag large holes in a river, to catch fish in a bay or even a shallow estuary, or in the surf.

For a 10-foot seine, I use ⅜-inch nylon rope for the top and bottom lengths. The doors should be made out of ¾-inch marine plywood. I use 2-liter plastic cola bottles for floats. The chain is good stout dog chain. Weight the bottom line with 4-ounce lead weights sewn right to the line. Experiment pulling this larger seine on the surface using a short towline and minimum weights to make sure it opens properly. Adjustments to the doors changing

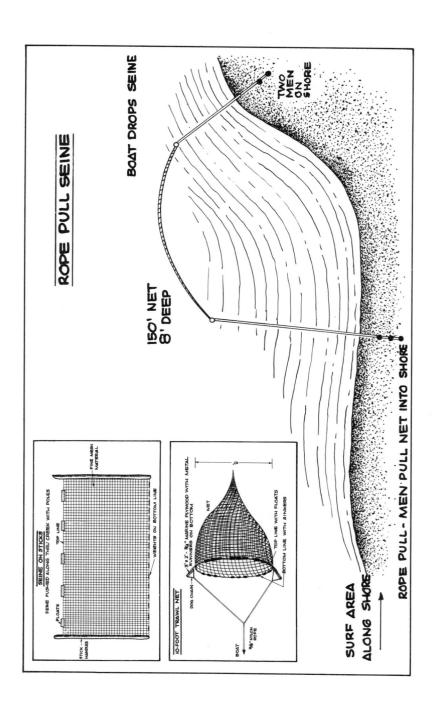

ROPE PULL SEINE

BOAT DROPS SEINE

150' NET 8' DEEP

TWO MEN ON SHORE

ROPE PULL - MEN PULL NET INTO SHORE

SURF AREA ALONG SHORE

SEINE ON STICKS

SEINE PUSHED ALONG THRU CREEK WITH POLES

FINE MESH MATERIAL

TOP LINE

WEIGHTS ON BOTTOM LINE

FLOATS

STICK HANDLES

10-FOOT TRAWL NET

3"x 2"x 3/4" MARINE PLYWOOD WITH METAL RUNNERS ON BOTTOM

10'

NET

TOP LINE WITH FLOATS

BOTTOM LINE WITH SINKERS

DOG CHAIN

BOAT

3/8" NYLON ROPE

the angle, or to the rope loop on the seine, may be necessary to
make it pull wide open.

It is very possible to salvage chicken wire, cloth, or netting to
make serviceable seines from. We have built seines many, many
times this way in the last forty years. But it's much easier to
purchase a seine ahead of time if it looks like one will be needed.

Making Nets

When the time comes, I will be willing and able to make any
reasonable-size net that I might need. Almost any small net can be
put together at home using miscellaneous found materials. The
real hitch is the time it takes to put them together. This can be
extremely time consuming.

Of all the nets one might build, the easiest start-from-scratch
type is probably the gill net. If one were to sit down and actually
knit a net, a gill net is probably the only one that could be finished
in an acceptable length of time.

Tools required are a net gauge, knife, and shuttle-line holder.

It takes a huge amount of line to knit a 3-foot gill net with 2-
inch mesh, 6 to 8 feet wide. Don't start unless the necessary materials are on hand. Limp, braided nylon line about the thickness of
15-pound monofilament works best. If not that, use linen string
and treat it with a solution of copper sulfate to keep it from rotting.

Freshwater gill nets in the 2- to 3-inch mesh class seem to catch
the most fish. This size also works very well for birds. Weights can
be fish sinkers or even lead globules cast in dry sand. Floats are
anything handy that are waterproof and buoyant.

I use a 3- or 4-foot gauge stick. Don't forget you are gauging to
the knot so the stick measures one-half. After making a few dozen
knots, the procedure will get easier and the product more uniform.

Describing how to knot a gill net is much more difficult than
actually doing it. Look at the accompanying drawing. The proce-
dures will be clear.

I make my gill nets in 4-foot sections hanging from the top line.
Three or four sections can be tied together to make a usable length
net. At first, the work will be slow and very sloppy. Not to worry,
however. It will still catch fish.

BUILDING A GILL NET

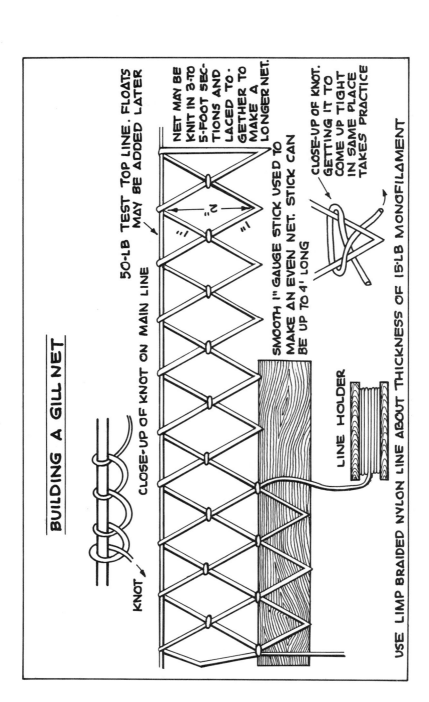

KNOT

CLOSE-UP OF KNOT ON MAIN LINE

50-LB TEST TOP LINE. FLOATS MAY BE ADDED LATER

NET MAY BE KNIT IN 3-TO 5-FOOT SECTIONS AND LACED TOGETHER TO MAKE A LONGER NET.

CLOSE-UP OF KNOT. GETTING IT TO COME UP TIGHT IN SAME PLACE TAKES PRACTICE

SMOOTH 1" GAUGE STICK USED TO MAKE AN EVEN NET. STICK CAN BE UP TO 4' LONG

LINE HOLDER

USE LIMP BRAIDED NYLON LINE ABOUT THICKNESS OF 15-LB MONOFILAMENT

Collecting Fowl

In an emergency situation, the second easiest meal to come by is birds. The fowl of the air can come from afar, reproduce rapidly, and are fairly easy to collect.

Bushel Basket Trap

One of my favorite upland bird traps is a little affair my Indian uncle used to refer to as a "bushel basket trap." Back in the old days when one could still find a woven-wood bushel basket, it was possible to use them to catch birds. Nowadays I make the enclosures out of ½-inch chicken wire on a light wood frame. Cover lightly with sticks, branches, grass, and leaves for camouflage. It is possible to construct the smaller traps out of medium-sized sticks if the wood is straight and uniform. The problem lies in trying to let enough light through the top and sides, without making the holes large and irregular.

Larger traps for turkeys are best built out of 3-inch diameter poles. Again, they must be straight and knot-free.

A pheasant/quail-sized trap should be about 3 feet on a side and 2 feet high. The best size turkey traps are at least 5 feet on a side and 3 feet high. Sometimes the captured birds jump around. The pen must therefore be held down with a stone or two on the top, or be made from heavy materials.

Pens are set out where the birds can be attracted in, using corn, sorghum, or other grain bait. Four trenches dug into the ground steer the birds into the trap. Upland birds will scratch around in the trenches looking for bait, and eventually work themselves under the trap. Once in the trench, they always try to get out through the top if they can see the light. That's why the top and sides of the pen must be fairly open with lots of light showing through. Loose leaves and other light duff scattered in the trenches and against the trap help. The birds busy themselves scratching and don't notice they are under the trap till it is too late. Birds you don't need for food can be released unharmed.

Gill-Net Bird Trap

A 4-foot piece of gill net can be stretched tight 4 to 8 inches above the ground, trapping birds in essentially the same way as the

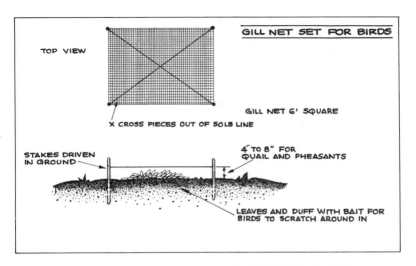

GILL NET SET FOR BIRDS

TOP VIEW

GILL NET 6' SQUARE

X CROSS PIECES OUT OF 50 LB LINE

STAKES DRIVEN IN GROUND

4" TO 8" FOR QUAIL AND PHEASANTS

LEAVES AND DUFF WITH BAIT FOR BIRDS TO SCRATCH AROUND IN

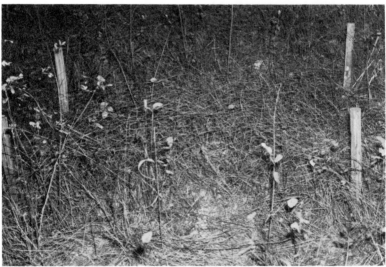

A gill net trap for upland game birds as used by the author. Diagram at top shows construction details. The beauty of this trap is that it can be made with any old piece of fishnet and four stakes, only taking a few minutes to set up. Grain is sprinkled under the net, and the birds crawl under the net to get at it. When they raise their heads, they are caught until the trapper returns for the harvest.

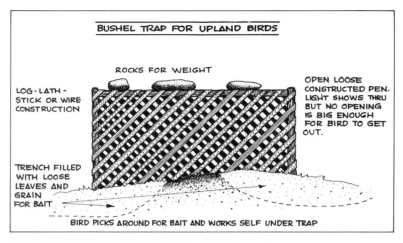

BUSHEL TRAP FOR UPLAND BIRDS

ROCKS FOR WEIGHT

LOG - LATH -
STICK OR WIRE
CONSTRUCTION

OPEN LOOSE
CONSTRUCTED PEN.
LIGHT SHOWS THRU
BUT NO OPENING
IS BIG ENOUGH
FOR BIRD TO GET
OUT.

TRENCH FILLED
WITH LOOSE
LEAVES AND
GRAIN
FOR BAIT

BIRD PICKS AROUND FOR BAIT AND WORKS SELF UNDER TRAP

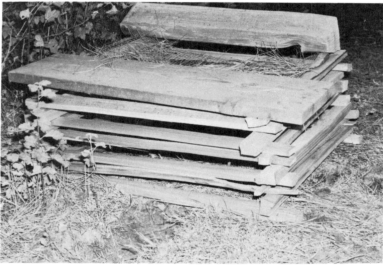

A pheasant bushel basket trap ready for action. This variation is made from split pine found in the area. One trench is dug under each side of the trap, with sorghum sprinkled in the grooves. Birds will eat their way under the trap and never think to crawl back out again. Trap should be heavy, since panicked birds will try to escape through slats.

bushel basket trap does. The birds work their way under this gill net trap while they are busy scratching for grain. When the pheasant or grouse sticks its head up for a look, it is caught.

Smaller birds like quail require a 1-inch net, set as low as 4 inches above the ground. Sometimes it is hard to keep the net taut. I either use two pieces of rope strung in an X between the opposing corner stakes, or use light chicken wire.

Ducks can be caught in a shallow marsh using a horizontal gill net trap. Stretch the net out about 2 inches above the surface of the water. Sprinkle corn or sorghum underneath for bait. The ducks will dive down into the shallow water, eat the corn, and come up into the net from the bottom. Most will stay right there, tangled. Again, chicken wire works very well here, perhaps better than gill net.

Duck/Geese Lines

Another desperation method of catching both ducks and geese that requires very little energy is to use fresh corn bait on a number 12 hook, tied up to 15-pound monofilament line. Set the rig with at least 10 feet of line attached to a 5-pound drag log unless no geese are working the area. A drag for ducks can be a pound or so.

Running Pheasant/Quail

A good healthy runner can, believe it or not, catch a pheasant or quail with his hands. I am not particularly healthy since I'm old, but using my Airedale I still do it occasionally. The theory here is that upland birds have very few blood vessels (hence the white breast meat) in their chest muscles. As a result they can fly only short distances before they become exhausted. Ducks have all dark meat and can fly hundreds of miles between resting times.

In fairly open, flat country, I will try to shoot a running pheasant with my .22 rifle. If I miss, it will often flush. My dog will then follow the flying bird and flush it again as soon as it lands. About half the time, the pheasant will head back in my general direction where I can run up and nab it. Don't try this trick with Hungarian partridge. They can fly back to Hungary before tiring out.

As an aside, pheasants are one of the easier birds to shoot on the wing with a .22, though in a survival situation I would never try sport hunting. I would, however, carry my rifle with me wherever I went. Then I could shoot any easy, big birds I saw along the road or by the spring.

Bird Snare Pole

Many birds can be caught with a wire snare on the end of a thin 6-foot pole. I have caught blue grouse, ruffed grouse, and francolin hens with a little snare on a pole. The main difficulty is getting close enough to the birds to loop the snare around their necks. Wherever quail or pheasants are abundant, they can at times be pinned down with a flashlight at night and snared in the same manner. This requires a good knowledge of the country and of game habits. Otherwise, there won't be a net gain in calories.

Guinea Hens

One of my favorite birds is the guinea hen. I intend to rely on them extensively during a prolonged emergency. Guineas are a kind of half-wild, half-tame bird that are ideal for people who will need some domestic stock to supplement their gardens and wild game. Guineas will make it just fine in roughly the southern half of the United States. Give them a modest amount of protection from the hawks and owls, a little feed now and then when it gets cold, and they will do wonders for the survivalist.

Originally guineas came from Africa. There are at least three different varieties in their homeland. In this country I have never encountered any but the small pearl types. They scratch around on the ground like chickens, yet roost high in trees like crows. When disturbed, guineas make a horrible racket. Some folks use them as an alarm system. Most important, they generally take care of themselves.

I harvest my guineas by snaring them when they come into the garden. That way I keep them out of the vegetables as well as keep their numbers down.

Guineas are getting harder and harder to find for sale. At one time every other farmer had some. The hatcheries still have them, but the price is high. It might be because other people have the same idea about using them.

Bird Flail

Here's one last method that I developed out of sheer desperation at a time when we were camping along the coast of British Columbia. It isn't a trap, being instead a bird flail of sorts. You may want to remember it yourself against the day of need.

Nine of us had been out in the coastal bush for almost two weeks. We didn't pack along much food and generally didn't require a great deal. The ocean was providing all our immediate needs. On the way back down the mountain to camp, I noticed a number of grouse and rabbits sitting along the logging road. Often they let us come within 10 or 12 feet. Naturally I thought perhaps I might be able to get some of these to volunteer to come home for dinner.

I cut a thin, dry cedar tree about 10 feet long and perhaps 3½ inches thick at the butt. Carefully I stripped all the branches off, leaving a clean stout pole.

Carefully and quietly I walked back up the logging road, holding the pole straight up in the air. Whenever I saw a rabbit or grouse, I inched up to within 10 feet of it, and slammed the pole down on the critter. Often I missed, but every now and then I did manage to brain one. Apparently they never saw the pole sticking straight up in the air. When the pole started to fall, it was too late. The only thing that saved them was my faulty aim. I clobbered enough in about forty minutes for everyone's dinner.

9. Survival Guns and Shooting

I realize full well that much has been written on the subject of survival guns. In most cases it is difficult to determine what qualifications most writers have that enable them to make credible comments. In many cases, it seems as though stock ownership in some of the larger firearms companies might be the first prerequisite.

Contrary to popular belief, it doesn't take many guns to survive. Bill Moreland's experience is proof of that. He didn't even have a .22 rifle for eleven years after he went into some of the roughest country in the forty-eight contiguous states. Bill learned early that he couldn't survive by hunting game—he had to trap it. Those who plan to wander around the woods hunting, rather than trapping, are in for a rude awakening.

Remember as well that Moreland avoided people. He didn't waste precious energy and ammo by getting in a firefight with the rangers!

The Wildman's example is the extreme. Owning a few more firearms is certainly a very good idea. Let it be known at the outset, though, that I am an advocate of a *few* guns and *lots* of ammunition.

Survival Gun Categories

Firearms for survival can be divided into two categories. Some overlap exists but generally there are those needed for military action, and those needed to forage with.

Unless you are going into the gun business in the next economy, one or two weapons each will be plenty for military purposes. If you are poor, there is no reason the same guns you hunt with won't make reasonably good defense weapons.

Of course, if you need an excuse to purchase more guns, by all means get one of the popular survival books and use it. The recommendations are broad enough that you could soon have a collection of 112 weapons of every kind and shape. About the only thing standing between the survivalist and all the guns his heart desires is money.

Military Rifles

In the chapter on equipment I mentioned that each of our women have a Colt AR-15. The men all have FN assault rifles, purchased years ago at a reasonable price. This goes along with my philosophy that the best military weapons are close to those the military in your area will use.

We just don't know which guns and ammo will be more available, so split the decision in favor of having some of each kind—.223 and .308.

Colt AR-15s are not particularly expensive. FN assault rifles, however, have appalling price tags. I still think they are the best shoulder weapon available in the world today. Yet to go out and buy them in today's market is unthinkable for all but the rich. There are too many other survival items that should have a higher acquisition priority.

Weapons held as strictly defensive in purpose should be reliable, rugged, of common military caliber, and be semiautos. Buying a military semiauto, as opposed to something like a Remington 742 or Winchester 100 even if they are in the right caliber, is important. Military weapons tend to be stronger, better built, of better design, and feature larger magazines. In addition they can be easily changed to full auto if need be.

Most survivors will probably not become part of a paramilitary police force, so they won't need to worry about the one or two machine guns that will be needed by groups like these. They can leave their guns semiauto and get along just fine.

The Heckler & Koch 91 is a super alternative to the FN. A neat little drop-in part available by mail converts them to full auto instantly. Be sure to buy no fewer than three extra magazines for each rifle.

Gun nuts these days spend a lot of time talking about how bad the AR-15 is, and what a puny cartridge the .223 is. Granted, the .223 is puny, but I did manage to kill a huge bear once with an AR-15; it took one shot right to the head. The bear weighed 415

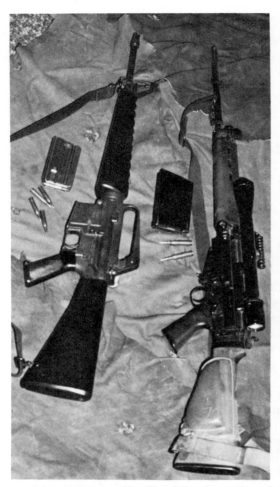
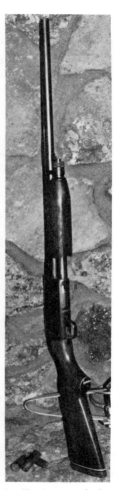

At left is an AR-15 in .223 caliber, belonging to the author's wife. At center is the author's own FN assault rifle in .308 caliber. Note its military scope and leather cheek pad. Both these weapons are ideal survival guns, due to their rugged designs, common calibers, and wide government usage. At right is an older model 37 Ithaca 12-gauge pump shotgun. A scattergun is useful for defense in the city, but small game will be taken with traps and snares, according to Benson's survival program.

pounds and squared 6 feet 5 inches. I have fired the same rifle over fourteen thousand times with little visible deterioration.

Some folks like the Mini-14. Where, pray tell, will you get parts for your nonmilitary weapon after the collapse?

If one is available, an M-14 would be a good choice. Needless to say, an M-14 is difficult and costly to come by. Presently our country does not have a commonly issued .308 long gun. Under a crashed economy or anarchy situation, there may not be anything but .223 weapons and ammo for us to procure. I suspect that the .308 would still be the best choice. It is a widely used cartridge throughout the world. Our machine guns are chambered for it. The problem in .308 will probably come from spare parts' unavailability and not the ammo. Those who have laid away a .308 should be able to get some ammo if they need it.

Some survivalists suggest storing Soviet bloc weapons such as the AK-47. Certainly this is excellent advice if you think that the greatest danger is from Russian invasion. I know from personal experience that it is nice to have weapons and ammo that are the same as the prevailing forces. In general the survivalists who advocate storing Soviet ammo and weapons expect more foreign military action than I see in the future.

Shotguns and Smg.'s

I have little use for a shotgun in a survival situation, outside of home defense in the city. During the seven months I worked in revolutionary Cuba, I carried a shotgun but never fired it once. In Africa I shot one perhaps a dozen times. All shots were at guinea hens running down paths. Our philosophy was that unless we could get five or more birds per shot, it wasn't worth the ammo. One time I shot a guinea on the wing. The boys were so surprised they almost fell over. They laughed about that for days.

I like the Ithaca Model 37 pump. It has a closed-action design, interchangeable barrels, is cheap, and has the most rugged extractor of any shotgun I know of. Ithaca 37s will shuck the lousiest reloads in and out with ease. My 37s have all had 26-inch improved cylinder barrels. They have been subjected to some of the worst sport hunting conditions imaginable and never failed. Pretty good for a gun that sells for a few hundred dollars, eh?

Some would-be survivalists have cached submachine guns. In my opinion, these can be a lot of fun, but have little practical value. If you want to have illegal firearms around, better to have a silencer for one of your game-shooting guns than an inaccurate, ammo-eating plaything. A silenced .22 rifle, for example, would be a fine survival tool.

Revolvers and Pistols

As with shotguns and submachine guns, I am not overly impressed with revolvers or pistols as survival weapons. We all have pistols, but they are not a priority item. There are a lot of survival items that should be purchased before a handgun.

When I was a kid I got a .22 single-shot pistol that I carried on a trap line. Pound for pound, it may still be the meat-gettingest gun in the house. On the surface, this may argue in favor of at least a .22 pistol as part of one's survival gear. The problem is that the vast majority of gun owners can't shoot a pistol worth sour grapes. They can't protect themselves with one, and they can't live on game shot with one. When the crash comes, there is no need to have another macho toy around that is nothing but an ammo burner.

Assuming you have accumulated most other survival items having a higher priority, you may still feel that you need a sidearm. As I said, we have some pistols, and can understand a person's motivation in this area. My recommendation is to stay with a simple .22 auto—a Ruger Standard Auto is a good example—and with a common military center-fire cartridge for the big pistol. Autos are much to be preferred over revolvers because of their reliability and ruggedness. Don't forget there isn't a country in the world that issues revolvers to its soldiers.

Since the U.S. now appears to be switching to 9mm for its issue sidearms, this leaves only one pistol in the big bore military class from which to choose. Everything else, as far as I am concerned, is second rate. My choice is the Browning HiPower. I am so prejudiced in favor of the HiPower that, to me, it seems the only pistol of this type worth having.

Hunting Rifles

The basic tool in most survivors' hunting arsenals should be a .22 rifle. At home I have a heavy-barreled Marlin Lever-Action with

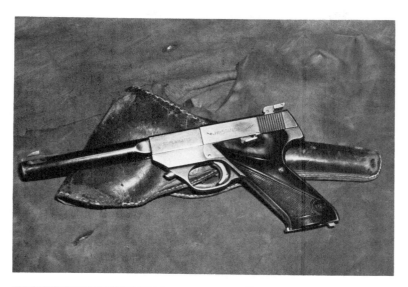

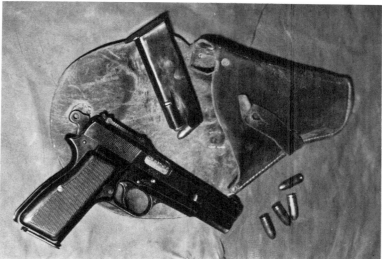

Top: A Hi-Standard Supermatic .22 semiauto pistol. Since pistols are often impractical in a survival situation, the author suggests waiting until all other supplies have been obtained before purchasing one.
Bottom: The author's Browning Hi-Power 9mm pistol. These pistols are reliable, accurate, have fourteen-round magazines, and use a common military round.

a four-power scope. The open sights are in a box in the gun cabinet where I can get them if need be.

Marlin levers are admittedly complex guns. Even so, mine will probably outlast me; but just in case, I have several single-shot rolling-block .22s in my caches, as detailed in the chapter on equipment. They provide insurance as well as some potential trading stock in the next economy.

Twenty-two rimfire cartridges are tough to reload. An adversary government or an economic collapse could completely cutoff manufacture. For that reason, I use another gun that is really my anchor small bore. It's a custom-made .25-20 single shot. This rifle is incredibly small, light, rugged, and accurate. Using cast bullets I can load up or down from 60 to 117 grains. The gun will shoot everything from rabbits to deer. It is quiet, the rounds buck the wind fairly well, and it has a much longer range than does a .22.

Aside from a good .22 rifle, the only other necessary hunting firearm for a survivor is a reliable, commercial bolt-action rifle in the prevailing military caliber. I like a Remington Model 700 or a Winchester Model 70 in .308 for this purpose. Put a good scope (probably four-power) on the gun and save the open sights. A good sling and swivel set are also recommended accessories for the bolt-action.

My principal game-shooting gun is a .338 Winchester mag Sako bolt with six-power Weaver scope. With it I can shoot through brush or across canyons. It will drop an elk at 600 yards like it was pole-axed. Under survival situations, this is a poor gun choice, though. It must be reloaded with brass and bullets that will be unavailable. When my cached supply is gone, I am out of business. A .338 uses lots of powder and is unnecessarily powerful in most survival situations.

At the present, it does the best job of dropping big game of any gun I have ever owned. It's just that when the crunch comes, I am certain it will be of little use.

Ammunition and Reloading

One of the agonizing questions all planners have to face is, "How much ammo or reloading supplies do I need to cache?" Ammunition, after all, is an Achilles' heel. I believe guns will

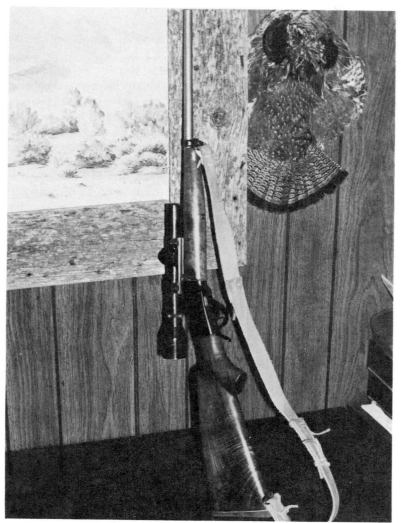

Ragnar Benson's favorite firearm: his trusty, custom .25-20 single-shot. It has downed everything from turkeys and coyotes to deer. This gun is light, quiet, and accurate. Cartridges can be reloaded for it in divers fashions at a lower cost than for other rifles suitable for larger game.

always be available to some extent. The premium items will be shootable ammo.

My personal recommendation is that you lay away enough ammo in your caches and in your supplies to last the rest of your life. I base this suggestion on the years that I have lived overseas in hostile situations, and on the past forty years that I have lived on what I shot or caught.

Fortunately, such an amount of ammo isn't all that much. You may be able to sell your TV for enough money to do the job. As I have tried to point out over and over, you won't be hunting your food in the next economy. You will, by and large, be trapping it.

Presently my family shoots about five deer and two elk a year. We do this with less than a box of shells. Twenty shells times twenty years equals 400. I therefore stored 1,000 bullets, primers, 10 pounds of powder, and 40 extra brass for my main rifle.

Two boxes of .22s are more than adequate per year. One hundred times 20 years is 2,000. We laid back 6,000 rounds. Still not a big item.

In my experience, those who try to suppress folks militarily have to bring guns and ammo with them. It then becomes nothing more than an academic exercise to figure out how to get the supplies away from the oppressor. Usually there is no shortage.

I figure 500 rounds per person per rifle as a minimum for the military weapons. This has always been enough in the past for me to start a program of ammo acquisition. Folks who live in the city may feel they need a bit more. Laying by 1,000 rounds rather than 500 is not that big a deal.

Yet 500 well-placed shots are one hell of a bunch. That many decomposing bodies lying around your retreat will kill you from pestilence if nothing else. If you plan to sit in an obvious castle loaded with food, a mini-gun and 60,000 rounds of ammo won't be enough to take care of the hungry mobs you could face. Hopefully you have figured out that your retreat must be hidden and unobtrusive.

My .25-20 is an economical workhorse; it gets about 1,000 rounds per pound of powder. I have laid back 10 pounds of powder, 5,000 small rifle primers, a bullet mold, 1,000 jacketed bullets, 250 empty cases, and a large quantity of lead.

Survivalists who are not gun nuts often assume the only place to buy ammo is at the local sporting goods store. They see prices like ten or twelve dollars a box, multiplied times ten boxes, and are scared off. The best place to get good ammo at reasonable prices is to buy surplus military rounds from the advertisers in *Shotgun News.* It will cost between one hundred twenty-five and two hundred dollars per thousand for even the commonest, most desirable rounds.

Improvised Reloading

While I was in Africa, I watched the natives filter nitrates out of cow manure to use in making black powder. Some may think it would be useful to include the process here; but folks, it just ain't practical. There are always better ways for reasonably intelligent people to get ammo than starting with cow shit.

Another trick the bush natives tried was to mix wood ashes from the fire with gasoline for use as a propellant in a pipe gun. The trigger was rigged to a hammer that struck a stick match in a hole in the barrel's receiver, something like a flintlock.

It was a miserable deal. The stuff had to be mixed fresh within five minutes of use, and then it wasn't very powerful. I am sure they got ten times as much game in their snares.

The English, who have extremely restrictive gun laws, use another trick to reload .22, 9mm, and .44 caliber *rimfire* cartridges.

The process is horribly time consuming, but it does work:

Thoroughly clean and dry the used brass. The inside rim should be brushed out to remove the old priming mixture.

New primer is made by cutting the heads off of "Strike Anywhere" matches, and soaking them in enough water to form a thin paste. Coat the inside rim of the clean brass with the paste. Allow the primer paste to dry thoroughly before continuing.

Use 43- to 50-grain cast bullets. Lyman makes several bullets that are designed for gas checks that will work. The best is the old Lyman #225353 plain-base mold which has been discontinued for years. Cast soft, and lube well if a gas-checked bullet is used. I use all bullets unsized.

Powder can be made by melting 1 cup of common household sugar in a steel double-boiler. As soon as it is melted—not dissolved—start cooling till the liquid can almost be handled. Stir in an equal volume of potassium chlorate and then let the mixture set up.

Next, fine-grind the white cake until it is small-granule powder. Fill the primed case up to the bullet area with powder.

Bullets can be held in the case without sizing by stippling the brass twice.

Most of the time the round will go off the first time. Power and accuracy are reasonably good. Be warned that this explosive mixture is extremely corrosive. Cleaning the firearm after each day's use is imperative. After four or five reloadings, the brass rims are too crushed to use again and must be discarded.

Ammo, powder, and primers that are sealed in airtight cache tubes will keep for many years. An adequate supply is not particularly costly. My final recommendation is to rationally plan your need for both guns and ammo and then start a program of acquisition. Initially it is better to buy more ammo. Leave the expensive, unnecessary guns for last, and your plan will work out well.

10. Big Game, Big Harvest

Depending on your circumstances, it may be a better idea to spend more time catching one big animal than exhausting yourself by chasing after small game. One deer or elk will last for months. A pheasant or duck might not last one meal.

The validity of this theory depends on the availability of game in your area. If small animals are all there is, then that's what you will have to go with. Just be aware that there are more big game animals around than most people realize. Several years back I did a little hobby project taking flash pictures at night of animals. I set out what was then a simple box camera and flash connected to a trip wire across a game trail. One of the pictures was of a huge bear. This was in a state park in north-central Illinois, a place where a friend bet me a hundred dollars that no bear had lived for fifty years!

Generally it is much less work for a knowledgeable woodsman to put up 100 pounds of deer than 100 pounds of woodchuck, snipe, or even carp. Deer, elk, moose, or bear can become a kind of staple, much like beef. Just don't give up on the little critters entirely. They break the monotony and many do have a special place in a survival economy. As an example, duck fat is the best snowshoe webb dressing available.

Defining Big Game

Big game is, in my estimation, anything that must be cut into smaller pieces and preserved. Elk, bear, moose, caribou, mountain goat, peccary, and deer all qualify under that definition. We won't cover them in this chapter, but larger salmon, sturgeon, muskellunge, and lake trout could also qualify here.

How Much at What Time?

One of the really important things our family has learned in the last forty years is how to estimate the quantity of wild game that we will need. You may take my word for the fact that more wild game exists than is generally supposed, but you still have to make accurate estimates of how much exists in your area. And you will have to know how much game your family will require and when it is best harvested. An overharvest, made imprudently at the wrong time, can be as serious as an underharvest.

There is a chance that there won't be enough game, big or small, to support you and your family in your area. This isn't the end of everything, if you find out now before the going gets really tough.

Assuming the deer we caught averaged between 95 and 120 pounds hog-dressed, and assuming deer were our only source of meat, our family of five would gobble down nine during our hungriest year. Two elk would work out to be one deer shy of doing the job for one year. Some folks tell me moose are larger than elk. I have caught quite a few of each and always found that they were pretty similar. It takes about as many of one as the other to live on. Caribou that I have taken have all been smaller than elk. In some cases, though, big old forest mule deer have every bit as much meat. Five big muleys would fill the bill for us.

The interesting eating occurs when the menu is a bit varied. As a general rule, I like to lay back five big deer, about seventy-five ducks, twenty geese, a few turkeys, perhaps sixty rabbits and squirrels, ten salmon, 150 trout, and fifty cod. Some years we get an elk or two, others it may be a moose. The fall bear that we invariably bag provides lard, and a quantity of chili meat.

If possible, I catch pike and walleyes, or bass, and store them rather than trout. We always count on some pheasants, quail, and grouse. The number varies from year to year. The important point is that the large animal, yielding hundreds of pounds of dressed meat, is always the anchor of our long-term diet. Without it the pickin's can get pretty lean.

Game Management

The economy of game management is such that a healthy, well-fed herd of twenty white-tailed deer annually will produce enough meat for one large family. Of the twenty, twelve will probably be does. Three of the does will be barren and should be harvested. Six of the bucks can easily be taken without harming the herd, leaving two bucks and nine does for breeding stock.

Next spring the nine does will probably have eight fawns. Four deer will have one fawn each and two will have twins. Three does will be barren. The herd's spring total will be eight fawns, nine does (three barren), and two bucks for a total one short of what we started with. If the winter is mild and/or the feed situation good, more of the does will twin and fewer will be barren. Often a net gain will result even if almost half the herd is harvested.

All of this requires a good handle on the game situation in your area to appreciate. Most people, including all of the average hunters, know only about 3 to 5 percent of the game in their areas, and that's all.

Moose can be cropped at a 25 percent annual rate, especially if you limit kills to bulls and barren cows. Thirty-five percent of the elk can be taken. Mule deer, however, are not as prolific as white-tails. Limit any kills to no more than one-third of the herd. This is acceptable since mule deer are roughly twice the size of whitetails. The only caribou I have hunted are the mountain type. I have no idea how fast they reproduce. Most folks, myself included, couldn't kill enough of these wary creatures to make a noticeable dent in their population.

Antelope are hardly in the category of big game. Most of the ones I have taken are about the size of a healthy billy goat. Better to raise the goats in the first place and avoid the hassle of looking for the antelopes. On the supply side, antelopes seem to cycle independently of any hunting pressure or seasons that I know of.

Bears breed every two years, but generally have twins. If you never take a bear with cubs, or one under about two hundred pounds, you will never hurt their breeding pool.

Selectivity

I am sure the next big question on everyone's mind is, "How does one go about being this selective when harvesting big game?"

To start with, all this selectivity is the ideal. It's a good target to shoot for but isn't always that practical. Usually the harvesting goal isn't even necessary unless you grossly violate nature's laws and kill mothers with young, for example.

Traps, by and large, are indiscriminate. They catch whatever happens by at the time. On the positive side, certain traps don't harm the animals. Inopportune catches can therefore be released.

Trap Lines and Harvesting Know-How

I believe the best method of making rational big game harvesting decisions in one's area requires running a trap line. I have known scores of trappers. Not one ever missed getting his year's worth of meat if he wanted it. There is something about the day-in-day-out routine that puts trappers intimately in touch with the outdoors. They walk the same paths, wade the same streams, look at the same thickets, and observe the same deer for weeks on end. Most important, trappers—even novice trappers—get used to looking for game and their signs.

Differences in feeding patterns, new tracks, new trails, use of salt, wallows in a spring, migrations, and other animal signs are all obvious to the trapper.

It's a whole different situation than grabbing a gun and heading out to hunt. Trappers are patient, observant, and quiet. Eventually they run across every animal in their territory, and know their numbers and habits as if they were part of the family (which in a sense they are).

Driving Deer

After a trap line, my second big game recommendation is that you learn to drive deer. Driving will work also to a limited degree on moose, elk, and bear.

The drives I am referring to are a maturing of the common surround-the-woods-and-march-through approach to deer hunting that one often sees in Pennsylvania, Michigan, and Wisconsin. Normally these drives rely on brute force using ten or more drivers to push the game through the woods to one of the many guns stationed on the other side.

Driving as we do it requires three or, at the most, four hunters who work together as a well-organized, well-trained team. The two or three who drive do so in a manner that allows them to push all the game in a given area past a hunter or two who have stationed themselves where they already know the game will cross. Usually there are no surprises. The hunters know how the drive will be made and who will get the shot at what time.

To be successful, driving teams must know the country extremely well, and be familiar with the likely pattern in which the game will move.

After a team understands this driving process, it is so easy to harvest deer, in particular, that hunters always wonder why they ever rambled around the woods aimlessly. Driving big game definitely produces a net gain in calories. It is a finding-collecting technique, not a hunting strategy. The biggest obstacle involves the fact that three or four similarly skilled, motivated people are required to pull off a drive. Sometimes that many are not available.

I work with my kids and several friends driving deer. In a survival situation we may not all be here. If that's the case other methods might be much more efficient.

The first thing a good driving team does is find out where the deer are staying. They do this by observing tracks, the deer themselves, noticing the timing of their migration pattern, new sources of food, or tracks on the common trails. The best advice is to drive only country that is known to contain game.

Initially, until they become good at it, drivers should push through an area with the wind, walking the country so the deer are scared up and moved out over predetermined paths. In this regard, the actual driving takes a great deal of skill.

Standers are every bit as important as drivers. It is imperative that they not be lazy. They have to learn to move silently without letting the deer smell, see, or hear them, around the drive area into position. This is incredibly more complex than the normal deer driver would ever suppose.

Driving deer is an art and not a science. For that reason, it is difficult to tell someone how to go about the process.

Deer Drive Check List

The following is a check list that will be helpful when driving deer with highly trained, highly motivated three- and four- man teams.

1. Give the standers plenty of time to get into position. Everyone on the drive should know where the standers will be and how the drivers will handle the terrain.

2. Practice first on smaller patches of woods. Drive them with the wind.

3. Stand where the game will come to when jumped. Learn this by observing how the game traveled last time you ran the patch, or what you saw running your trap line in the area.

4. Drive open areas faster than bushy spots. Patiently standing with the wind at your back will run even the smartest old buck out of a dense thicket.

5. Be prepared. Novice drivers are often surprised to find the game leaving as much as half a mile ahead of them.

6. Know where your partners are at all times.

7. Take the high ground whenever possible, but don't neglect to break through brushy draws or tangled thickets if the deer are using them.

8. Lazy drivers are worthless. It takes work to do the job correctly.

9. Don't be bashful about driving a woods on a bias. Run it any way that pushes the animals out.

10. Take advantage of natural terrain, cover, streams, and lakes.

11. Practice until your team is good at it.

Snaring Big Game

My next choice for collecting big game in an emergency would be to use snares. Refer to the chapter, "Snares and Deadfalls," for complete information on making and using big game snares.

Relative to any other method of taking big game, snares are often the easiest. It is certainly easier to learn to snare than to drive big game. The biggest drawback lies in the fact that snares are sometimes indiscriminate. This isn't totally true. Some adjustments can be made, but generally you have minimal control over what you catch. It is possible to set a larger loop, avoiding the smaller deer, for example. Or set the loop higher off the ground in places where a heavier concentration of bucks is known to exist. Loop size for deer should be from 13 to 18 inches in diameter. The bottom of the wire is set about 30 inches off the ground, depending on the type of deer you are after.

Coastal blacktails and whitetails are easy to snare. Mule deer are tough to impossible unless they are concentrated by bad weather.

Other Emergency Big Game Traps

There are several other traps and methods that work well for big game. Some are completely natural and others are manmade.

When I was poor "hayseed" in my teens, we used to burn the grass off a local bayou every fall. The burning process was good for the ecosystem of the marsh. It allowed new growth to come up the next spring, without adding a layer of vegetation that would have eventually choked out the open water. More important at the time, we were able to run a number of deer out past standers with rifles. Usually we were able to pick out a couple of nice bucks for the larder. Under normal circumstances it was virtually impossible to run the deer clear of that heavy, tangly cover.

Another good natural trap that comes to mind is one we found accidentally along a reservoir. I had just made an unusually long shot at a deer. The round hit too far back, and the buck ran off badly wounded. We tracked it in the six-inch snow for about five hundred yards. By that time it had zigzagged onto a wide peninsula jutting out in the water. The area comprised perhaps sixty acres. Small pines and thick scrub brush covered the rolling ground.

Three of us lined up and quietly drove the area. The wind was at our backs so the best we hoped for was to move the wounded deer out into the open at the water's edge.

The drive wasn't twelve steps old when we heard splashing. The cover was high enough to block our view, so we couldn't be sure. It sounded like our game had broken cover and was trying to swim for it. We quickened our pace.

Much to our surprise, there was a lot of additional splashing. Anticipating that the deer might be headed back to shore, we ran down to the water's edge. There, out in the water, were four deer.

One was obviously dead, which we brought into shore. Three others were swimming for land perhaps a hundred yards away. It wouldn't have been very hard to shoot the swimmers. Our wounded deer had apparently died of shock when the cold water hit its exposed intestines.

This peninsula isn't the only natural deer trap I have run into. It is the best, however. Others include a small canyon, a little woods near an orchard, and a weed patch in the middle of a large field.

Pen Trap

A good pen trap for deer and elk can be made using three tiers of wire fencing. I got the idea years ago from a Fish and Game Commission trap that was then used to live-trap elk.

We built ours out of old 48-inch high stock fence strung on 12-foot tall poles and trees. The pen was open in the front and back to make the deer (in this case) less suspicious. It was triangular in shape, about 35 feet long on a side. I put some bags of salt in the trap for bait.

In three or four months, whitetails were coming into the pen every few days for a lick of salt.

Finally I closed one opening in the trap permanently, and over the other rigged a piece of fence nailed to a log frame. Using a trip-stick trigger similar to the one shown in the "Snares and Deadfalls" chapter, I was able to fix a falling door that looked like it might work. The deer had to go into the trap and mill around a bit to hit the trip, which I thought they would do if they came to the trap in the first place.

It was about a month after hunting season when the deer started coming into the trap. Finally one hit the trigger, trapping three. There was a doe and fawn and a spike buck. We kept the buck since our family was generally hard up for a meal back then.

Nothing came the rest of the season.

The next fall, we set the trap again, but only got one buck. The pen trap wasn't tremendously successful, but it wasn't that bad, either.

Bear Traps

Bears are best caught in nail can traps, or in the heavy 5/32-inch snares I covered previously.

Nail can bear traps are large versions of the coon spike trap described in the chapter on "Small Permanent Traps." They are made out of four pieces of ¼-inch boiler plate (6" w. x 12" h.) and 20-penny nails. Construction is just like that of the smaller spike trap, but on a larger scale. Bait is either honey, sardines, or peanut butter.

Bear snares are quite effective, relatively easy to set, and cheap. I like to build a small pen out of 12-inch logs if I can't find a natural place for the snare. The idea is to set up a path the bear will have to travel to get at the bait.

Use a sapling spring pole with a breakaway line. Attach the snare to a long drag rather than attempting to fasten it permanently. The bear will push into the snare and trip the spring pole, which will snub up the wire on his leg. In turn, the bear will fight the snare, pulling it off the spring pole, but not the drag log. By then the noose is tight. All Mr. Bruin can do is drag the log around, leaving a trail wherever he goes.

Dogs

People who know how to handle hunting dogs can do well with them on big game forays. The pooch becomes a sort of roving, semicontrolled driver. Many dogs will track deer but few hunters know how to take advantage of that fact. This is because they don't know where the deer is headed, or how to get around to the likely deer crossing area in a timely manner. So these folks don't know the game, the territory, or their dogs.

The best dogs are ones that trail rather slowly, barking often. Deer are more fearful of a fast-moving dog that only barks occasionally.

Big Game Yards

In the middle of a bad winter, deer, elk, moose, and almost any big game will group together in protected areas. Eastern hunters call these places "yards." Westerners simply refer to a canyon or draw where the game has "migrated." Under these conditions, the critters can be practicably hunted. It still takes some skill. You will have to come in upwind, quietly—still a far cry from bumbling around the woods with a gun.

Don't harvest these animals late in the season unless it is an absolute emergency. The rough weather drains their body fat. Often they become poor tasting and rank.

Rather than wandering around the woods aimlessly, I find yards in spring while looking for mushrooms. Dead deer, deep worn trails, and tree bark eaten up to a height of six feet are sure signs the game wintered there.

Nets

In many places in the world, nets are used to catch big game. Some Africans build giant elaborate rigs stretching several hundred yards. The animals are driven out of the bush into the closure where they are run down and killed. Rather than being enmeshed in the net, they are actually trapped in an enclosure.

Most African game is able to jump quite well, and could easily bound right over the trap. The natives mitigate this problem by hiding and camouflaging the net so the game runs into it before realizing that the barrier is there. Once it hits the net, the natives are johnny-on-the-spot to grab it.

In England, large enclosures were set up that looked much like huge trawl nets stranded on the land. Deer were driven into these pockets and killed by the lord of the manor, with a sword.

People in this country generally think of animal nets as being dropped from the skies onto unsuspecting animals. This, of course, is unworkable, and nets are seldom set up for big game.

The best method I know of using nets here is one that people on Vancouver Island use to collect coastal blacktail deer. It requires a large piece of old seine in the 2- to 4-inch mesh class. They set the net up on a well-used game trail, strung across the path so it forms a walking barrier. Initially the net is anchored right on the ground. It then rises up farther down the path to a height of about 4 feet and finally tapers off again down to ground level.

The deer run up the path, bounding into the net which tangles on their feet. Instead of backing out, they continue in till all feet are off the ground, and all they can do is roll around and fight the webbing.

Many times the Vancouver Island nets are used in conjunction with organized drives.

Drags

Mention was made of using log drags in snares to slow big game up enough so the trapper can follow their trails and get to them. The same principal is valid in a number of different applications.

Most of us remember the tales of the Eskimos who used a seal stomach filled with air as a floating drag on a harpoon line to catch big whales.

A bleach bottle on a line will wear out lake trout and bring them up, even if the line is relatively light.

Floating drags also work well on speared sturgeon, which are native to some of the large rivers out west. Normally these fish have great strength (they can also weigh up to 1,000 pounds!). A drag on the end of a medium-weight line with a float will bring them up nicely after they have swum and struggled until exhausted. With a drag like this, it isn't necessary to use giant spears and heavy ropes that often fail in actual use.

Beavers can often be speared from a boat at twilight as they move about their ponds. Some beavers can get up to sixty or more pounds and are very difficult to horse-in using brute force alone. In the past I have been successful with a 2-foot line with a gallon bleach bottle as a drag. The beaver seldom swam over fifty yards. Keep the floating drag in mind for use on any large fish or other animal that must be brought in from deep water.

In conclusion, any two of these emergency survival methods will harvest all the big game one family can use. Obviously, some are more applicable in some areas than others, yet all are fairly universal in their application. They can provide you with the means of using nature's livestock to survive.

11. City Survival

If our government falls, the big cities will soon destroy themselves. Public services will end. Panic will set in, with rioting, looting, and burning soon to follow. Death may be everywhere. After the cities are in ruins, criminal gangs will attempt to migrate to the country where they will continue their ugly business in more fruitful territory.

At that time the now basically uninhabited city may be a boon to the determined, prepared survivalist who has managed to stay there discreetly. He will have the entire city, its contents and growing game population to himself. There will be abundant fuel, building materials, machinery, and tools, and a million other items that the guy in his country retreat must have either stored or go without. The cities will be a scrounger's paradise. In time, a brisk trade may develop between the country folks and the city dwellers, in pre-twentieth century style.

Whenever people are left to their own inventions, some damn incredible things occur. By far and away, humans are the most resourceful creatures on earth. In Africa, Europe, the Near East, and Asia I have seen some truly inspired products of human ingenuity—shoe factories way back in the bush, fish catching co-ops twenty-two hours by road from the nearest electricity, people manufacturing modern machine guns with hand tools, chemical plants, garden tool factories, and so on. Wherever government is absent, and people can put together some kind of system to protect their property, there will be an innovative explosion.

One item has weighed heavily while putting this book together. I realize full well that relatively few people who are serious about survival can afford the romantic, adventurous approach most authorities suggest. We can't leave the city for a secluded retreat in the hinterlands. What would we do for jobs and an income there? We need our jobs to survive *today*. Without paying work, none of us could ever hope to start a caching program, or buy any needed

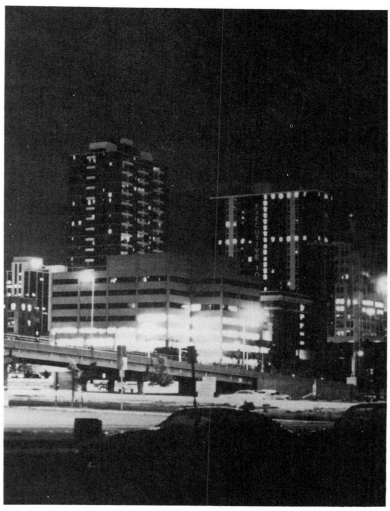

Living through a collapse presents a great challenge to the urban survivalist, but it can be done. Advance preparation is the order of the day here. Besides storing away extra survival supplies, the urban dweller must scout the city for unassuming, yet defensible living quarters, areas that will make good garden patches, and sources for water. At this time, small game should also be located. This includes finding pigeon roosts, squirrel trees, fishponds in parks, and any trails habitually used by rabbits, squirrels, or other city critters.

survival gear. I am fairly well-off, but I can't afford two homes, or even an adequate city home and a crummy country retreat. Readers who make sixty thousand dollars a year or more, or who have relatives who live in the country, might be able to put together a hideaway. But for you and me, the idea of a retreat, unless it is very modest, is pie-in-the-sky dreaming.

The supposition I make, then, is that most of us will have to live in the larger cities till the collapse. Keep in mind that most of our country's populace is concentrated in a relatively few urban areas. A few will escape to the country, but most of us will continue to survive where we are now.

The good news regarding all of this is that it *can* be done. I have survived in the city for several years, and so can you. Essentially all I am suggesting is that you can keep your job, live where you do now, and in addition, give up six hours of TV per week to start learning and preparing for your future survival.

Caches and Supplies

First of all, folks who know they will have to make it in the city should store extra food to supply them during the time right after the initial collapse. There should also be additional provisions for self-defense.

I believe, for instance, that people who are of the Mormon religion are going to have a rough time in the cities. Almost everyone knows that these folks store a one to three years' supply of food as part of their religious obligation. I predict that after the collapse, organized mobs will seek out the membership lists of the various LDS stakes and attempt to appropriate the food these people have laid away. Probably some interesting firefights will ensue, since Mormons certainly aren't pansies.

Very few buildings in the city are fortified enough to withstand the frontal assault of a determined, violent mob. It is better by far for the survivor to be discreet. Don't broadcast the fact that you are caching for survival. Keep your stores and your caching places to yourself. Then, after the collapse if someone comes around, it will be a random scavenger who can be more easily dissuaded.

My recommendation is that you plan for the worst, and cache or store enough provisions to last six months. This means enough food to live on without leaving home.

If you have enough money for gourmet niceties, that's fine. Otherwise, I am talking about stashing a hundred pounds of beans, a sack or three of rice, five pounds of baking soda, a couple of additional bags of flour, and so on. Sit down and figure out what you will need. The simpler basic foods are not costly.

Defense in the city will be a close-range situation. Hunting, the other use for guns, will for the most part be limited to small game. Whenever I have lived in the city, I have used my .22 bolt-action rifle far more than any other gun. My recommendation, then, is to double the number of .22s you store—not a particularly expensive proposition, especially compared to buying a retreat on two acres in the mountains.

Other than extra food and some additional .22 ammo, your cache/supply program will probably look much like the guy's in the country. Like the supermarket basket of goods, everyone's situation will be different, requiring a different mix of items.

After the first six months are taken care of, give some thought to how much will be needed during the next year and a half. Assume you will be able to raise or catch half of your needs during that time. Then lay aside yet another supply to get by while you are rebuilding your life.

Water

In the city, one of the toughest commodities to come up with will be water. Needless to say, it's not going to come out of the tap like it did before. You should develop a contingency plan now for acquiring your water later.

Some suggestions include digging a well, driving a one-inch pipe for a well, collecting rainwater on the roof or with a plastic sheet using a cistern, reprocessing water, desalting water, and getting it from a lake, river, or pond.

Howard Ruff suggests providing a waterbed for every member of the family, which is not a bad idea if you also have a method of purifying the water. A family of four might have up to two thousand gallons in waterbed storage. If all the water was saved for drinking and cooking, it would last a good long time.

Should your inventory show that you will need to drive a well, or haul water from a creek, collect it off the roof or whatever, start now putting together the special equipment you'll need.

Collecting Game in Town

There are great numbers of wild game in most cities. Having heard me say this a number of times, you will probably start looking around and eventually agree with me. Other than the downtown core areas, I don't believe food will be a serious long-run problem for the intelligent survivor. As more and more people depart the cities, the game population will literally explode. Some of the animals might be ex-pets, but they will be nutritious and filling.

Cities that I have observed which collapsed for one reason or another all had thriving populations of dogs. This was true for almost all of them except where the population was predominantly Islamic. After a bit, the inhabitants got hungry enough and started to try to shoot or trap the canines. Undoubtedly most people would do the same.

As an aside, I have spent too many hours hunting gone-wild domestic dogs. The challenge is intense. Wild dogs possess an intuitive knowledge of man's limitations, with none of the apprehension that one normally associates with coyotes or wolves. Dogs will come right into your yard without fear. But if a human is detected, they are gone like smoke in the wind.

A good way to collect dogs requires that you put a female in a pen that has three number 2 steel traps connected to 20-pound drags around it. If the bitch is well into heat, the traps won't even have to be camouflaged.

Dogs that are hungry are a bit easier to bring in to bait and trap. They are still elusive, however. Set snares in their runs if you can locate them.

The following is a proven gourmet recipe for dogs. Some parts of the formula may not be possible for the survivor, since it is designed to taste good. The point is that some not-so-desirable animals can be fairly good table fare if one overlooks the origin of the *piece de resistance.*

Roast Leg of Dog

Take one medium 25-pound dog (dressed and skinned) and separate both hindquarters from the carcass. Set the balance of the meat aside for later use in stew.

Take a long pronged fork and pierce the meat over and over until it is tender. Heavily salt with tenderizer if available. Rub in and allow to rest at least one hour.

Rinse in water and lemon juice. If the latter is not available, thoroughly wash in clean water.

Marinate overnight in the following if available:

2 cups burgundy
¾ cup olive oil
2 cloves garlic
dash of hickory salt
½ teaspoon nutmeg
10 peppercorns

Next day, preheat oven to 350 degrees Fahrenheit. Remove legs from marinade and arrange in a glass baking dish, underside up. Slice meat to bone along the bone. Layer with bacon, cover dish, and bake for sixty minutes.

Remove from oven and let cool. While cooling, stew ten medium tomatoes.

When cool enough to handle, arrange dog legs on platter, mix bacon with tomatoes and arrange around the legs on the platter. Fill the slits with your favorite legumes. Sprinkle with parmesan cheese.

Bake again for fifteen minutes and serve.

Obviously this is intended to be a tasty recipe for meat that is otherwise unacceptable to many people. In a survival situation, some of the ingredients may be hopelessly impossible to come up with.

Most Common City "Game"

Another abundant creature in the cities is the rat. I should have mentioned rats first, but the thought of eating a rat is worse than chowing down on a dog; at least for me it is. The Chinese eat rats with relish. My experience in China was such that I am convinced these people do as well as they do because they use all of their available resources to the best of their ability. But I still don't like the idea of eating rats.

A few years ago the *National Geographic* magazine published an article on common rats. The story pointed out that rats are one of the most persistently prolific groups of mammals in the world. They breed in great numbers in some of the most hostile circumstances that can be imagined. The point of the article, and my point as well, is that rats will always be with us. In that regard, they are probably the most certain food sources available to the city survivalist.

Surprisingly enough, if it weren't for their incredible numbers, rats would be classed as a difficult animal to collect. Some of the big ones are also feisty and mean as snakes. In sewers and dumps where they thrive, they can often be "spotted" at night with a light, and shot. This can be the easiest way of getting a great number of them.

Rats regularly use the same runs, and can be trapped or snared. Use a number 1½ trap or a copper wire snare. The trap need be only slightly hidden. Usually so many travel the runs that eventually one will get caught. If there are a lot of other rats around, they will eat the ensnared individual unless you check the trap regularly.

Baited box traps catch rats well. If the need is great enough, you probably could set out three traps and catch three rats a day in a big city for the rest of your life.

Smoking the dens dug in and around buildings and empty lots will drive rats out where they can be shot. Water poured in the dens will also chase them out. I kill them with a .22 this way now for sport. Later it may be a deadly serious business.

Hoards of rats can be caught in a barrel trap. The trap is built out of an old steel drum. Weld or bolt three hinges on the top of the barrel and fasten 1-by-4-inch boards to them. Counterweight the boards with lead weights so that a slight weight shift will tip the board into the barrel.

Bait the ends of the board with small pieces of meat stapled to the ends within the barrel. Most of the time these rigs are used with a foot of water in the bottom so the rats will drown. Where they are abundant, rats will soon fill the barrel.

Cats as Catch Can

Readers who have stuck with it through my discussion of using dogs and rats for food may have predicted my next city-survival food topic: cats. I should make it clear that I cringe when thinking about eating any of these three types of critters. The point is that

BARREL TRAP USED FOR RATS
(FLOATING VARIATION MAY BE USED FOR MUSKRATS ¿ TURTLES)

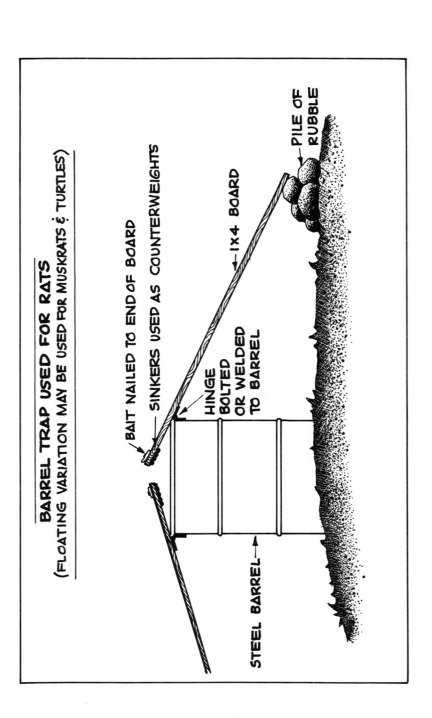

BAIT NAILED TO END OF BOARD

SINKERS USED AS COUNTERWEIGHTS

← 1×4 BOARD

PILE OF RUBBLE

HINGE
BOLTED
OR WELDED
TO BARREL

STEEL BARREL →

they are the likeliest source of easy nourishment in the scenario I envision. When you need to fill your belly or else, rats, cats, and dogs will start to look mighty appetizing indeed.

U.S. cities are home to large numbers of house cats. I have never eaten one myself, but have partaken of the loins of a cougar. It was quite good. A house cat would be similar in taste, I think. Use the trusty "Roast Leg of Dog" recipe if necessary.

House cats are easy to catch in a box trap baited with a mouse or some smelly fish. Don't bother trying to conceal the trap; cats just don't care. City cats, like all other animals, have their favorite haunts and runs. Set some snares for them in this case. Cats don't mind one bit poking their heads through a snare loop.

City Birds

Another common creature in many cities is the pigeon. They are prolific and have the added ability to range far and wide for food. Look in old buildings with a second story entrance for their roosts. The birds like to get inside someplace high that they can leave from without having to fly to gain a lot of altitude. Also look in barns, under bridges, the eaves of houses, building ledges and cornices, around statues, in parks, etcetera. One of the best ways I know of to find a batch of pigeons is following the circling flock to their roost at dusk.

Pigeons can be attracted in with grain bait and caught in copper wire snares. At night they can be spotlighted on their roost and caught by hand. When we were kids we captured literally thousands of birds this way. Sometimes they are up too high in the buildings and must be shot off their perch. A .22 works nicely for this, the only question being the propriety of using a valuable .22 to collect four ounces or less of meat.

Pigeon eggs are edible, if taken from the nest early and collected regularly after that. In some locations there are enough pigeons to make this egg business worthwhile.

City Squirrels

Most cities harbor large populations of tree squirrels. Whenever I lived in the larger metropolitan areas, I made extensive use of these guys. Several times when we were poor I got so I couldn't look a squirrel in the eye. Sometimes we had them to eat more than once a day—roasted, fried, in pie, and cut up in stew.

While I was working on this book, my brother reminded me that he took quite a few squirrels in town with slingshots. I still prefer to shoot them with CB caps (down-loaded .22 rimfire ammo). True enough, my brother did become proficient at collecting squirrels with a slingshot. It can be done, and is an option to keep in mind.

Aside from slingshots and .22s, squirrels are easy to catch with box traps or tree snares. A steel trap set up in a favorite tree also works. Hackberry, buckeye, hickory, walnut, and oak are all good bait trees.

Box traps for squirrels should be baited with nuts, bread, or a piece of fruit if available. Usually box traps work best at times when food is scarce, such as during winter or fall when the nut trees aren't bearing fruit.

Some fairly nice jackets, gloves, and vests can be made from squirrel skins. Feeding yourself on squirrels will produce a substantial number of skins as a byproduct. Be sure to save every one.

Pulling Rabbits . . .

Rabbits in many cities are practically a domestic animal, besides being the tastiest item on our urban survival menu so far. They have lived so long around people that they've lost most of their fear of us. The major predators for city rabbits are domestic dogs and cats. In the western city where I live now, there is a very strict leash law, allowing the rabbits to proliferate to the saturation point.

I like to use box traps with bait for rabbits, or catch them with snares. Steel traps set in runs work okay, but often mangle the rabbits. Traps should be set in brushy areas where you have previously noticed rabbits, or other signs of their presence, such as droppings.

Rabbits have a limited range. This means the city rabbit you see was probably born within a one-block radius of where you saw him. Therefore if you catch too many rabbits, you will wipe out the breeding stock. Squirrels, on the other hand, forage over long distances. Several different times we have tried to catch as many squirrels as possible and never affected the observed population.

Exotic Wild Game in Town

During the times I have lived in cities, I've always been surprised at the number and kinds of open-country wild game that has made its home there. We regularly caught pheasants, quail, gophers, coons, possums, muskrats, ducks, geese, and even an occasional mink. One southern town I lived in had a thriving population of grey fox as well as some skunks and groundhogs.

By far and away the most common animals in city suburbs with mature trees are coons and possums. These are very good animals for readers to know about because of their size and the fact that they breed rapidly. City coons and possums are expert at living around people without being seen. On the other hand I have usually been able to trap these fellows quite easily. They are used to human scent, steel, and tracks that would scare their wild cousins right out of the county.

Whenever you suspect that one of these animals might be in your area, set out a box trap baited with a mouse, peanut butter, or a piece of dried fish. Box traps are especially good in these circumstances. They remain operational over long periods of time and when they do catch an animal, it is held inconspicuously out of sight.

Occasionally coons and possums will work garbage cans, dumpsters, nut trees, and fruit orchards in town. Whenever you observe this happening, set out a steel trap. Check the trap often so it and the catch won't be stolen.

Pheasants and quail can be shot in town with a .22 or trapped. Use a basket trap or some snares to get them. Quail, especially, are very small. Don't fool around for days at a time trying to pick up one or two of these birds. There are only three ounces of meat, at best, on a quail.

Muskrats live commonly around lakes and ponds right in town. My bet is that if you have a park with a pond in your town, there are muskrats in the pond; and further, that somebody is trapping them now, just to keep the numbers down. After the collapse, you can take on this trapping job. Muskrat numbers can expand very quickly, creating a meat and fur source for the city survivalist who has his head screwed on right.

Folks who are new to the survival business often ask how they can be sure that muskrats live in the ponds near them. If the pond has reed grass or cattails growing in it, the rats may build a grass house much like a small beaver lodge. However, they often live in burrows dug under the bank. You can spot the tunnels leading out where they exit underwater along shore. Where there are a lot of muskrats, the bank will cave in and there will be holes where the den's chambers used to be. The earthworks look a lot like common rat diggings.

Muskrats are easily caught in small steel traps set in runs about three inches deep in the water. A better method is to build a floating barrel trap. Very few people will recognize the barrel for what it is. It will catch a number of muskrats at once and will keep right on producing up till the time the water freezes over.

To build a floating barrel trap, take a good, solid 55-gallon steel drum with ends intact, and cut out an opening one-third of the way down from the top in the center of one end. Now weld or bolt two hinges in the opening and fasten 1-by-4-inch boards on the hinges. Weight the boards with fish sinkers so they tip easily into the barrel. Put some rocks in the barrel so it sinks to within 2½ inches of the opening. Simply allow the trap to float in the pond. Check it every couple of days or whenever the bait gets stale. I like apples, carrots, or corn for bait here.

These same ponds that harbor muskrats attract ducks. Be ready spring and fall to either shoot or trap the fowl as they migrate through. If you aren't sure when they might arrive, rig some number 12 hooks on monofilament line attached to a log. Bait with corn and throw it in your pond. Ducks passing through will eat the corn and catch themselves, signaling the fact that more ducks will soon arrive.

City Fish Ponds

Don't forget that fish live in most of the ponds found in cities. Be prepared to start catching these guys in large numbers. Fish soup made out of the lowly carp may not sound good now, but later it might be all there is.

While you are checking out the available ponds and rivers, be sure to look for turtles and crayfish. Sometimes the best way to tell if a big old snapper inhabits a pond is to set out a turtle line. Take a two-foot piece of flexible wire. Number 16 brass wire is the best. Tie it to a number 2 hook. Bait it with a solid chunk of smelly bait and tie it to a root with fifty-pound line. Rebait the hook every morning. If you don't get a turtle in a week or so and the weather has been good and warm, there probably aren't any around. Large ponds in city parks sometimes have a large turtle population. If you get one or two, you may want to set a turtle trap to increase the rate of harvest. Turtle traps are either floating barrel sets baited with meat or are oversized fish traps, with funnels large enough to let the turtle in. See chapter 6 for plans.

Raising an Urban Garden

Cities are good places to raise gardens. (See chapter 12.) Even in the core areas there are vacant lots, terraces, parks, and other open areas where food can be raised.

Two or three years after the collapse, large regional gardens may come into being. An enterprising person may dig up an entire park, or a series of eight front yards, and actually start a small farm. This would happen only if some kind of property rights were reestablished.

In the meantime, be sure you survey your neighborhood for potential garden sites. Experiment raising some of the survival vegetables mentioned, and then start a seed storage program for the kinds you know you will need. Don't forget to lay aside all the tools you will need, including spare handles for rakes, shovels, and hoes.

Fruit and Nut Trees

It isn't practical to plant nut trees for use after the collapse. We will need them long before they have time to mature. Better to snoop around your neighborhood and find mature nut trees that could produce survival rations during the time of need.

On the other hand, it is practical for city people to plant dwarf fruit trees. Under normal circumstances they will produce in three to five years. The mature trees require very little space and are not particularly tough to grow. An average apple or plum tree will yield no less than three bushels of fruit per year. Four of them would go a long way toward making the winter less long and cold.

Some early spring day, after you have identified the fruit trees in your area, take a small saw and pruning shears, and go out and prune the trees you know about. Cut out all the old dead branches.

Trim the outside branches back. Take out some of the center limbs so you can reach the fruit, and the light can get in.

Continue cutting till you have a single, lower tree, devoid of suckers and long branches. Many wild trees require an incredible amount of pruning. It may help to look at a properly cared-for tree in a commercial orchard, or one at the home of a friend or acquaintance.

Sweets in Town

The summer of 1947 I moved off the farm into a suburb of Chicago. My wife and I rented a small house in an older section of town. Most of the houses were bunched up on small lots. Out on the parkways there were a number of large trees, so huge they shaded over the street in many cases.

Quite a few of these trees were big old elms that died years later of Dutch elm disease. The thing that really surprised me was the fact that probably one-third of the trees were giant old maples, exactly the same kind that Uncle and I had tapped for maple sugar on the farm. I was glassy-eyed. Anyone with a similar collection of maples would have been rich in my previous economy.

I went down to the salvage yard and bought a total of almost twenty feet of miscellaneous length ½-inch galvanized pipe, to make syrup taps from. At home I cleaned the scale out of the pipes and cut them into 8-inch pieces. Using a hacksaw, I eventually split all of the sections in half, giving me a total of about fifty pipe halves. Three inches in from the end I drilled a ¼-inch hole through the bottom of the pipe half. The last operation was to file a notch in the pipe to hold a bucket handle.

If all of this seems complex, refer to the illustration on page 151. The tap is very simple, as the drawing shows.

Using a brace and ⅞-inch bit, I drilled holes 3½ inches deep, five feet off the ground in the surrounding maple trees. Most of the neighbors let me put taps in their trees. Some out in the parkway had to be tapped at night. Trees three feet in diameter got one tap, the four-foot ones two, and some monstrous trees got three.

I drove the half-pipe taps into the tree till the hole just matched the cambian layer in the maple. It was a crude system, but it worked quite well. I used some clean gallon buckets hung on the spigot to collect the sap. Starting about the middle of March, we got about twenty gallons a day for three weeks.

Maple syrup should be boiled slowly in a very large cast iron pot. The heat should be distributed evenly. We didn't have a cast iron pot so used an old copper washtub over an ancient gas stove that was originally put in the basement to heat wash water.

Maple sap boils down at the rate of about forty to one, depending on how thick you want it when it's done. We got almost ten gallons out of my effort. I gave four gallons away and my wife canned the remainder. Six gallons is more maple syrup than the average family uses in a year.

Survivors should be ready to tap maple trees if need be. They are a good source of a very scarce item.

Another source of sweets for city dwellers is from honeybees. Domestic bees are easily kept in towns and suburbs. Survivalists who live where they can make it work could start raising bees now. Many a backyard in suburbia could be the place of residence for docile varieties of honeybees, especially if the yard is closed off by a high hedge or fence that the neighbors can't see through.

During the early sixties, we lived in a medium-sized town in Iowa that suffered incredibly when a killer tornado came through. Many of the big old elms, maples, and oaks were so torn up that it took three days to clear a path through the place. After the cleanup started, there were so many chain saws running all over town that it was impossible to carry on a conversation.

One of the handicaps the cleanup crews faced was the hostility of the many colonies of bees that were disturbed in the holocaust. The number was truly amazing. Apparently the weaker, hollow trees or those with hollow limbs blew down first. It seemed as though every fifth hollow tree had bees.

As a result of that experience, I started to look for bees in the city. Using the techniques described in the chapter on bees, I was able to locate probably twenty-five wild colonies in ten years. It was far more fruitful to hunt them in the city than in the country, at least at that time.

Two problems did arise. People in small towns often raise bees. Many times I spent valuable time tracking bees to commercial hives. Another problem arises after the wild bees are located. Often it is impossible to cut the tree or otherwise harvest the honey once it is found. In a pure survival situation, this would not pose a great problem.

Most people don't have the bucks to live in both a city and a rural environment. Often we survivalists think of the folly of someone coming from the city to live in the country when they have enough money to do so.

On the other hand, after the insurrection has burned itself out cities will be good places to scrounge needed supplies. The survivors who make it will undoubtedly be the scroungers—people who know how to make it in *any* environment. Just remember, if you have to stay in the city, give yourself the benefit of some preparation. Practice, so you can be ready when the time comes. Your situation is far from hopeless.

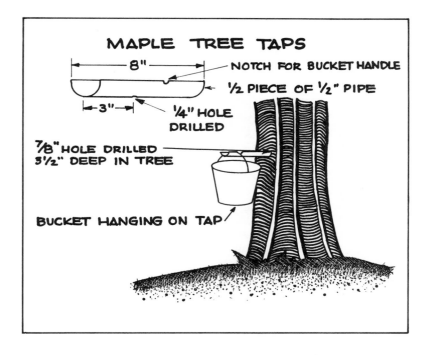

12. Edible Plants and Survival Gardening

A few minutes' research at my local bookstore indicates that there are already plenty of books devoted to the subject of eating plants that grow wild in the outdoors. Most such books go on and on about all of the neat edibles you can find in the bush, if only you know what to look for.

Well, I know from day-to-day experience what to look for out in the wild and, believe me, it isn't budding Canadian thistle. First and foremost, we should remember that the native Indians who lived where you and I do today did not subsist on wild plants. They ate some of them to be sure, but their most important sources of food came from game and cultivated crops. Contrary to popular belief, the Indians did not wander around the woods casually picking this and that to feed their faces.

This does not mean we should abandon our original plan to study the indigenous Indians to see what they lived on, only that we should try to find out if they raised corn, yams, or whatever for a significant portion of their diet.

Secondly, we must understand that a lot of wild vegetable products taste pretty bad. A few years back I lived where camas roots were common. We often dug and ate them. All of us agreed they were pretty good. So are wild rice, acorn meal, buckeye biscuits, dandelions, and even cattail roots. Some of the other stuff—thistles, skunk cabbage, ferns, and tree bark—is terrible. Even if I could find enough to live on, I wouldn't. There simply is no reason to live in such misery.

My solution is to make use of an extensive, intelligent garden.

Gardens make a lot of sense, today and in the future. Correctly done, they entail little work. More important, a garden will pay for itself five times over as compared to a similar amount of store-

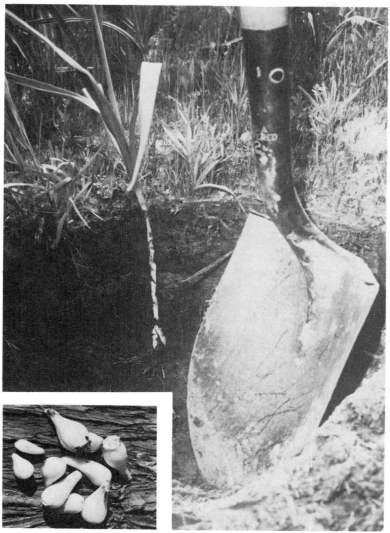

Camas roots are one type of wild plant that is nutritious *and* good-tasting. They are most commonly found in the West. Plant tops look somewhat like onion leaves, with blue or white flowers. Best time to dig them is during spring, but be sure to leave a healthy patch of plants undisturbed, so they'll grow back next year. At center of main photo is an exposed camas root during digging. Inset photo at left shows camas roots close-up. They can be boiled or roasted, and taste like a cross between a potato and an onion.

bought groceries. In the process, you will be acquiring an invaluable skill that will help keep your family healthy.

City Gardens

City residents often talk about how hard it is to raise garden patches in their areas. I honestly believe good, productive patches of vegetables can be produced even by people living in core area apartments.

At least that was always the case when I lived in the city. At one time we had potatoes and red beets growing in the grassy area around an interchange. My wife raised tomatoes and lettuce in a window box, and I talked the maintenance man into letting me raise a few sugar peas in the flower beds. We didn't raise all the vegetables we ate, but we didn't work that hard at it, either.

People who live in suburbia or on the outskirts of larger cities have it made. There are hundreds of acres of parkways, front and backyards, parks, median strips, grass interchange dividers, and other open spaces that will support gardens. My prediction is that most of these plots, especially front and backyards in suburbia, will be dug up for gardens someday.

In the USSR, 4 percent of the tillable land provides almost 50 percent of the nation's food. This is the land privately held and farmed, as opposed to the remaining 96 percent which is in collectives.

Survivors located in the cities will, in my opinion, have plenty of space on which to raise gardens. At times it may be necessary to hide the plot, yet the space will be there. A lot of vegetables look like weeds and are easy to hide. Obviously, raising these varieties will be important for the survivor who doesn't want his spuds stolen.

The following is not a complete unabridged treatise on gardening. The emphasis is on efficiency and practicalities. That means easy growing, large yields, and good storability are my principal criteria. Of these, storability has to be the most important. As you may know, tomatoes are easy to grow in many places. But how does one store them for more than a week or two? We pick our tomato vines and hang them in the root cellar. The tomatoes ripen nicely over a period of about four months.

Carrots

The principal advantage of carrots is the ease with which they can be grown under a wide range of conditions, and their long storage life.

In a root cellar they will keep for two months, and refrigerated carrots last four months. I have never fooled with either method. Left in the garden and covered with straw, leaves, or dead grass, carrots make it through the winter just fine. It seems kind of ridiculous to go out and shovel off the snow in January to get at them, but that's what happens. Carrots will keep through early May anyplace in America, with the exception of the Deep South where it gets quite warm and they turn soft. But the growing season there is so long it doesn't really matter. By the time the old carrots spoil, the new ones are almost ready to be harvested.

Under southern conditions, survivors should plan to plant carrots very early in the year, and again late in fall. The result is a steady supply all year long.

Scatter the tiny carrot seeds in a thin line about an inch deep in the ground. Often the planting will be too thick. They can be thinned easily enough after they come up. This wastes seed, however, and is unnecessary. Better to thinly scatter the seed in the first place.

Many people don't know carrots when they see them growing. Seed scattering, rather than planting in rows, will attract little attention along a roadside or in a flower bed. Four rows of carrots 35 feet long will provide one-third of all the vegetables a family of five will need for an entire year.

Spinach

The second best vegetable for the survivor is spinach. It meets the criteria of easy growing under a wide range of conditions, and good storability. Spinach tastes all right when cooked, but we use most of ours as leafy greens in salads.

Spinach grows just about anyplace in the U.S. In the warmer climates, it should be started very early or grown over winter.

Covered with straw or similar material, spinach will last all winter. We pick ours in the snow. It won't grow new leaves so it must be left in fairly lush condition in the fall.

Scattered around, the plants look like weeds and won't be bothered by other people.

Plant two rows 35 feet long for five people. Work up the ground well and plant about 1 inch deep in fine soil.

Squash

To successfully raise squash, the reader should start to figure out now what varieties do best in his area. The variety question is a big one since there are so many different types to choose from. As a general rule, squash are sensitive to cold weather. Varieties exist that thrive one place but do poorly in others. Some do very well even where the summer is short and cloudy.

Squash offer a big advantage in the storability department. In a root cellar they will last seven months. I have kept them in my basement sitting on the floor in a wooden box for five months.

Seeds from squash do not store well. The answer here is to save some seed each year for planting the following year. If a year is missed, fertility will decline about 40 percent during the second year. Under those conditions, plant 40 percent more seeds.

Plant squash in mounds, about eight seeds per mound, after all danger of frost and cold weather has passed. The mounds should be 6 feet or more apart. Squash plants and fruit are obvious, making them a poor choice for a clandestine garden.

We have never been able to eat the production from eight hills of squash by ourselves. Some of these monster veggies get up to fifteen or more pounds each, and there can easily be ten on a vine!

Asparagus

In much of this country, asparagus grows more like a weed than a tame crop. If not a weed, it propagates like one. Asparagus grows naturally in fence rows, along highways, in vacant lots, in the lawn, and just about anyplace.

Asparagus will not do well in sour forest soils, very infertile soils, or where it is shaded. All of these constraints are easy to overcome. I have raised asparagus in a northern Michigan sandy pine forest by cutting the trees around the patch, and planting the crop in a 2-foot bed of horse manure.

Asparagus is started from roots either purchased or dug from a wild patch. Plant the roots 2 feet apart. Twenty-five roots will yield enough asparagus to feed a family of five.

From a survivalist's standpoint, the problem occurs trying to store asparagus. It will keep up to four weeks in a root cellar. Otherwise it must be frozen or canned. The ease with which it can be grown more than offsets this weakness.

Red Beets

Beets pass all of the aforementioned criteria with flying colors. They are easy to raise, easy to store, hard to detect growing semi-wild, and truly provide a large amount of food.

Red beets like cold weather. They should be planted early in the North, or in fall south of the Mason-Dixon line. Be sure to spread the seeds out in the row when planting to avoid the need for thinning.

Storage is best handled similarly to carrots. Beets won't last through a severe northern winter in the ground, but they will stay in fairly good condition until the middle of January.

An added advantage to red beets is the fact that the plant tops make good eating. At least they are better than going out and gnawing on trees. We like them cooked with a vinegar sprinkle.

Only an astute gardener will recognize beets growing at random in a vacant lot or weedy front yard.

Red beet seeds keep reasonably well in sealed containers. Their shelf life is estimated to be about five years.

Corn

Corn is modestly difficult to grow some places in the U.S. In the southern two-thirds, it grows very well if enough water can be applied, and if the insects don't get it. Readers who are not familiar with farming or gardening are going to be shocked at how much insect pests cut crop yields. Without insecticides we could not possibly feed the present number of people in this country.

Corn is sensitive to the many climatic and soil variations throughout the country. For this reason, thousands of corn varieties have been developed that are each suited to a particular range of local conditions.

My recommendation is to find out what varieties the local farmers are growing, and buy a bushel of that seed for storage. A bushel of corn seed will keep a family in corn for fifteen years. Fortunately the seed will easily keep twice that long.

Seed must be reserved because commercial corn is a hybrid. The kernels can't be saved and replanted the next year.

By now the more astute ones among you will have recognized the fact that I am recommending field corn and not sweet or garden corn. There is a difference.

Sweet corn tastes better, but that's its only plus. It yields far less, germinates poorly, is more sensitive to frost or droughts, and doesn't keep nearly as well.

Other than the high yields, the best reason to raise corn is that the finished product will keep for decades. It requires no special drying, refrigeration, root cellars, or treatment. The toughest job will be keeping the mice and rats out of it.

Corn, in my estimation, is one of the best long-term emergency foods. It is far better than wheat, which has lower yields per acre, about the same food value, and takes considerably more equipment and time to harvest.

Corn should be planted about 9 inches apart, 2 inches deep, in rows 36 inches apart. The soil must be well worked to a depth of not less than 12 inches. Plant only after the ground warms up and all danger of frost has passed.

Twenty rows of field corn 35 feet long will feed a family of five for no less than four months. Corn can be ground, baked, made into cakes, soaked in water, stewed, or carried in a sack on long journeys.

Corn was one of the primary food sources for the Indians. If you are serious about living off the land, you will develop your corn raising skills now.

Potatoes

Perhaps potatoes are a good bet for survivors. They grow nicely under a variety of conditions, yield well, and keep fairly well in storage.

I don't presently plant potatoes because of the work involved harvesting them. Two people can sometimes spend as much as one day digging and bagging 500 pounds of the blasted things.

Also, potatoes are started with sets. One freshly cut potato chunk with no fewer than two eyes is planted per hill. Under most circumstances it takes one pretty good-sized potato for every two hills. The yield will be about ten potatoes per plant.

Potatoes do well in fertile, well-drained soil. They must be rotated into new ground every two years or disease will start to be a problem. Live potato plants are easily hidden. In fall the tops die, making the hills tough to find without prior knowledge of their location.

Even in root cellars, storage can sometimes be a hassle. Many times spuds dug in September will be sprouted by Christmas. In dry climates they can be left underground where they grew, over fairly severe winters. So readers who are worried about food looters can leave the crop hidden in the mounds.

Twenty mounds produce two hundred pounds of potatoes under all but the most adverse conditions. That's enough to make a year's supply of stew for the average family if other vegetables are available.

Lettuce

Leaf lettuce can't be stored, so it isn't really a survival garden item. The reason I mention it is because lettuce is easy to grow, good tasting, and nutritious.

Plant either very early or very late in the year. A few feet of ground seeded every three weeks will provide a large quantity of good eating.

In the southern half of the U.S., lettuce can be grown year-round.

Peas

Pod peas can be a pain in the neck if they are handled incorrectly.

Plant peas as a winter crop in the South and very early in the spring in the North. They provide good eating for six months or more. After they dry on the vine, they can be stored almost indefinitely.

Pea seeds keep well from year to year. Just take a few out of your food store for planting.

The real work involved with raising peas comes when you shell the fresh green peas out of the pods. Rather than doing that, we eat the peas, pods and all, till they are two-thirds mature. After that, we let them dry, later using the dried, shelled peas in stew and soup. Dried peas are much easier to pick and shell than fresh peas.

Five 35-foot rows of peas take care of our family for a year. Obviously, they aren't all we eat. Yet pea soup is still one of our favorites. We have it about once a week.

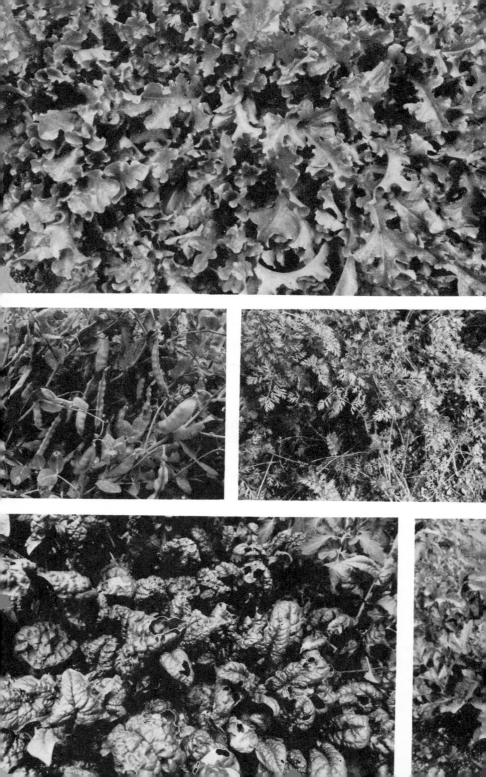

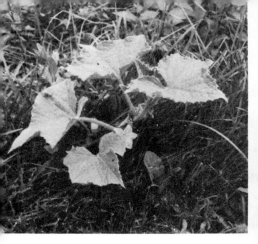

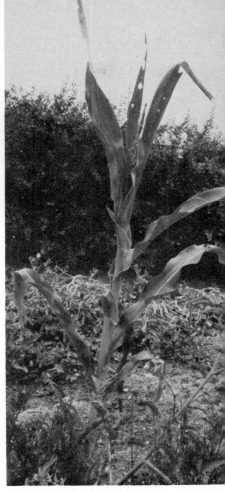

Selection of hardy, well-tended plants in a survival garden located in the Rocky Mountains (*bottom right*). City survivalists should keep in mind plants like carrots (*left*) and potatoes (*bottom center*). They are hard to distinguish from weeds, easy to care for, and store well. Veggies like peas (*left center*) dry readily on the vine, and keep in storage for years. Lettuce (*top left*) can't be stored, but is a great summer treat. Not only does squash (*top center*) store for months, its seeds can be saved and used again next year. Benson advises growing feed corn (*top right*) instead of sweeter varieties. Sweet corn is difficult to dry and store. A healthy stand of spinach (*bottom left*) rounds out this survival garden.

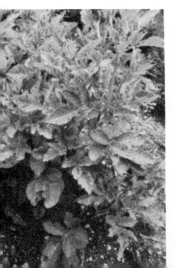

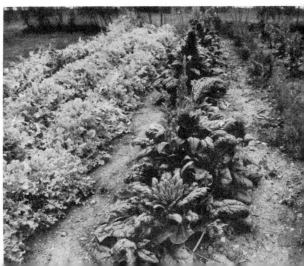

Kale

Kale is a hardy, easily grown vegetable that produces lots of food and grows all over the U.S. It can't be stored except if frozen or canned, which isn't particularly important. The plants are practically perennials. They bear good leaf crops all winter long except in the northern quarter of the U.S.

Most people won't recognize kale when they see it. The seeds store and germinate very well.

The only problem I know of with kale is the taste. I like it stewed with potatoes. Other people can't stand it—probably the same people who talk about eating grasshoppers and nettles!

Zucchini

Zucchini is what is known as summer squash. It grows and produces much faster than other varieties that mature late in the fall after the first frost.

The advantages of zucchini lie in the ease with which it can be grown over a wide range of climates and soil types, and its generous early yields. The disadvantage is the fact that zucchini must either be frozen or canned within a few weeks of harvesting.

People in general seem to know what zucchini looks like. The vines grow on top of the ground in plain sight, bearing fruit where all can see it. In that regard it may not make good survival fare if the owner is forced to plant in vacant lots, median strips, or parkways where others might help themselves.

Sometimes the production of just a few hills of zucchini squash can be overwhelming. The wife of a close friend put in twelve hills a few years back and harvested thousands of pounds of squash. She was a frugal person who hated to throw anything away. Soon she was out of neighbors, friends, and business associates who wanted zucchini. Still the flow continued.

When I asked her why she didn't just plant two or three hills, she told me that she and her husband had been transferred around quite a bit by his company. The last place they lived, zucchini did rather poorly, she said. Apparently the bugs got many of the small plants.

After that episode, her husband started rationing the zucchini seed.

Obviously, there are a few more considerations to raising a survival garden than just the question, "Will it grow in my area?" Factors such as storage, hideability, and versatility are also important. Again, my recommendation, especially for those of you who will have to survive in town, is to spend a few hours now learning what will grow and store in your area.

Storing Seeds

Perhaps half of the garden vegetables that are commonly grown are hybrids. As a practical matter, this means that it isn't possible to use seeds saved from some of these vegetables for next year's crop. Resulting growth will reflect the various crosses. Most of the produce will be tasteless, spindly, and weak.

It used to be possible to make general pronouncements as to which vegetables were likely to be hybrids and which were not. This is virtually impossible any longer. Many seed packs don't even give this information.

In a true large-scale survival scenario we would most likely revert to using the same seed for replanting as the Indians did. If all we have is hybrid seed, the results will be mixed, until we can begin to develop some nonhybrid varieties.

Squash seeds are quite often not hybrids. We have saved them at home for years and years. Some of the varieties we use today might be descended from original stock. To keep squash seeds, separate them from the pulpy core material and dry. Be careful the seeds don't mold.

Carrots may not go to seed under any circumstances in some of the colder areas of the U.S. To produce seeds, the roots must be left in the ground over winter. A deep freeze can easily kill them. People living in the southern half of the U.S. will find the seed stalk set by early winter. Others might get seed the following spring. Most carrots are hybrids that will revert to crummy, wild-looking produce after the first year anyway.

Spinach and kale go to seed the second year unless the leaves are closely cropped. Usually, but not always, the seeds are not hybrids. Harvest is made by rasping the dried pods between the palms of the hands and blowing the chaff off.

Red beets and lettuce go to seed the first year in most places. Save seed and try. In many cases the produce is acceptable. Be sure the seeds are dry before attempting to harvest and clean them.

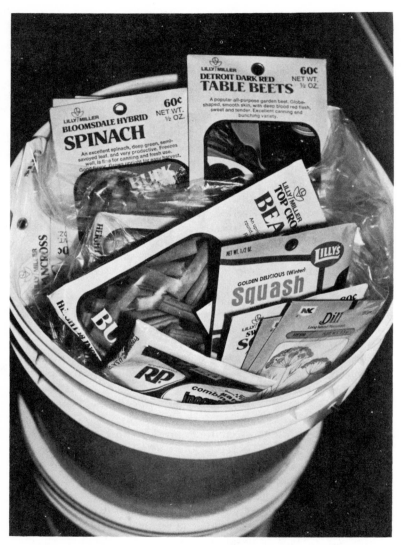

A 5-gallon restaurant bucket filled with a selection of garden and herb seeds. Survivalists will have to determine which vegetables grow best in their areas. For optimum storage, seal all seeds in airtight buckets kept in a root cellar, if possible. Seeds should be replaced and used every few years.

Peas are merely dried and set aside for use the following year. Usually they will produce a good crop even if they are hybrids.

I didn't mention beans as a survival garden crop in the first section because they flunk some of the important tests. They are, for instance, very visible. Everybody knows what beans are when he sees them growing. No sense, I believe, in planting a crop for someone else to pick. Also, beans are tough to keep green unless frozen or canned. When they dry, harvesting is a lot of work and the resulting yield relatively small.

On the plus side, many bean varieties are not hybrids. They will breed true year after year from saved seed. Beans are also quite easy to grow.

Take your pick. Maybe beans should be in your survival supplies. The seeds keep for many years.

Most garden seeds will keep well for seven to ten years. The exceptions are lettuce and carrots which keep for three years at the most. Lettuce, for the most part, is not hybridized, so collecting seed each year isn't a problem. Many carrots are hybridized. This presents a dilemma. You can't store the seed and you can't collect them for next year.

I recommend storing garden seeds in sealed plastic buckets that are kept in the root cellar or the basement. By so doing, two crucial requirements are met. The seeds stay consistently cool in a dark place, and they keep dry. Dryness is very important. Folks living in damp climates should hang the seed container over the stove a few days to be sure the seeds are bone-dry before storing.

Being careful about storage pays dividends. Carrots that normally have a shelf life of two years had a 40 percent germination rate after three years when we planted them one spring.

Right now garden seeds are cheap. Fifty dollars will buy enough to last for ten years. Store plenty of seeds, especially vegetables like corn, peas, carrots, and spinach.

Fruit Trees

During the last five or six years fruit trees have mushroomed in price. On the average their prices have about tripled, as demand far outstripped supply.

There is no way of knowing for sure, but it seems likely that many homeowners are planting a fruit tree in the backyard as an extra food source. Apparently these people realize that a healthy fruit tree or two can supply dozens of bushels of produce.

For instance, apple trees bear so much fruit during some years that they cover the ground below with a rotting, stinking layer of wasted fruit. The mess is so onerous that municipalities will not plant fruit trees on public property anymore. Logically we should be planting something that provides food, rather than being strictly ornamental. Logic may again prevail in this country—who knows?

There are large numbers of wild fruit trees growing around this land. Some, like pawpaw trees, are strictly wild, never having been domesticated. But most are old, gone-wild fruit trees that could bear again if properly cared for.

Serious readers should get out and locate all of the fruit trees near their homes and retreats. A little pruning and care will often pay off handsomely.

Basically there are two types of fruit trees available at your local nursery: dwarf and semidwarf. Most full-sized trees seem to have passed from the scene. The larger trees are used by commercial orchard owners who have lots of room for big trees. Homeowners' demand probably isn't great for the big trees, explaining the scarcity of the channels you and I would normally use.

Survivalists planting trees as a future food source should plant the largest variety that space and availability will permit. Bigger trees bear more fruit, are more winter hardy, survive insect blight and other pests better, and live a lot longer.

Fruit trees are planted in late fall or early spring when they are dormant. Dig a hole three times the size of the root ball at least twice as deep as needed. Half-fill the hole with dirt mixed one-to-one with peat moss, chopped leaves, grass and straw, or any other organic material. Place the tree in the hole and cover the roots with finely divided topsoil. Water right after planting and regularly during the growing season.

New trees must be pruned to the point that the root growth about matches the top growth. Ask your nurseryman to do this job and to explain what he is doing.

Fruit trees usually bear well after the fifth year. Some may start earlier in some parts of the country, but don't count on it. First yields are always very small. This is the most persuasive argument

I know of for getting out now and planting food trees. Even if they are slow-growing ornamental nut trees, do it now.

Conditions vary from area to area, so it is tough to recommend specific varieties of fruit. For me to tell you to run out and buy a Lodi apple tree as opposed to a Red Delicious is folly. Assuming you have no idea what to plant, can't find a good book on the subject, and have no friends with fruit trees in the backyard that you can check out, I recommend the following. Drive to a small town that has a large garden supply store that has been in business for a number of years. People in big cities usually can find a place like that located near the oldest, largest suburb. Go there on a Monday early in the season before the rush starts. Explain what you are doing, and nine times out of ten you will get very good advice. If that's impossible, get a Sears Farm & Ranch catalog and order from it. Be very wary of most of the mail-order supply houses. They sell largely ornamental shrubs and trees. Often the fruit trees they have are junk and/or are delivered in poor condition.

My preference is not to raise pears. They keep poorly—although they can be dried. Our crew doesn't like the taste which is the real reason there isn't a pear in our orchard.

Peaches are another fruit that keeps poorly. Nevertheless, there are several peach trees in our yard. The harvest comes in much sooner when it's nice to get some variety, and we really like the taste. Peaches also make excellent fruit leather.

Peach trees bear after only three or four years, but are often dead of old age at ten. In some regions of North America they have to be sprayed continually or the yield will be poor and wormy. On the plus side, some amazing new varieties of peach have been developed that produce fine fruit even in colder areas like Montana and Minnesota.

There are two kinds of apples: summer and winter varieties. The summer apples keep poorly but are a welcome change early in the season when they mature. We use our summer apples to make applesauce, fruit leather, and other recipes. Yields of summer apples are often three times larger than winter varieties. Check first, however. Some climates are so hostile that summer apples won't grow.

Bright red winter apples will keep five months in a root cellar. When I was a kid we normally harvested about five barrels of apples that we stored in our root cellar. During the winter Dad would open the cellar on warm days and get out what we needed, including a peck or two of apples. The only problem with Dad's approach was that, instead of just grabbing out a bucket full, he would always pick the ones that were going bad. Thus, it was guaranteed that we would never eat a truly good apple for at least five months!

My recommendation is to plant three winter apple trees and one summer variety, provided you have enough space. That much fruit will more than take care of your family, assuming someone who also covets your apples doesn't organize an armed attack on them (more on this later).

Cherries won't keep using normal storage techniques. Like so much other fruit, they are awfully good eating at harvest or if they can be canned or frozen. Otherwise it's a feast or famine situation.

Don't plant cherry trees if space is scarce. They require a male and female tree, one of which bears little fruit. Sour cherries self-pollinate so require only one tree. Hopefully things will never be so bad that I shall have to live on sour cherries. Be warned that some people have a tough time raising cherry trees. The damn things die on them consistently for no apparent reason.

Plums require little work, are fairly consistent producers throughout the U.S., and can be dried for long storage. Modern varieties really taste good, too. Wherever I have lived, I have planted plum trees with favorable results. They take up little room for as much fruit as they produce. Raise the more sugary type of plums for dehydration purposes.

Pruning Fruit Trees

Fruit trees must be pruned to yield well. There is definitely an art involved in pruning trees that will have to be at least partially learned by survivalists.

Here are some simple rules to start with:
- Always remove all of the dead branches.
- Never prune a cherry tree unless the branches are dead.
- always make cuts on live branches immediately ahead of a bud unless, of course, the whole branch is taken.

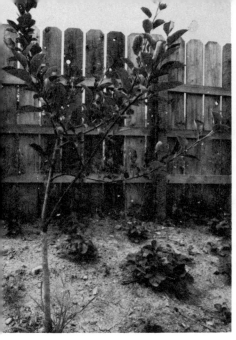
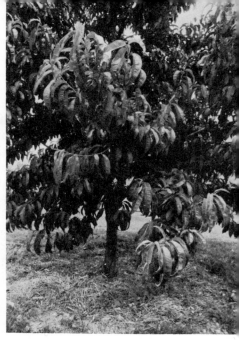

Four different dwarf fruit trees, all about five years old and just beginning to bear fruit. Jonathan apple tree (*top left*) provides a harvest that can be stored in a root cellar through January. Fruit from a peach tree (*top right*), cherry tree (*bottom left*), and plum tree (*bottom right*) won't keep for more than a few weeks. It is either canned or made into fruit leather.

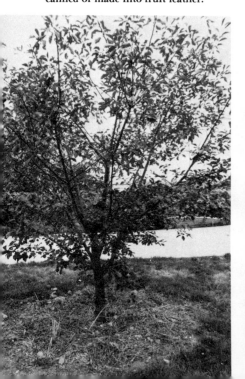
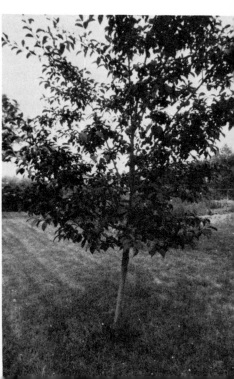

● Prune peach trees very lightly early in spring. Take a few, weak internal branches each year and let it go at that.

● The object of pruning is to open the tree up to sunlight and to restrict the growth. Otherwise the tree may produce a half-ton of one-inch wormy fruit.

● Apple trees should be heavily pruned during the dormant season. Leave five or six evenly spaced branches and whack the rest off. Amateurs usually don't prune apple trees enough. Get the majority of the shoots out of the tree.

● The inside branches of plum trees should be removed during the dormant season. Some light pruning on the new growth should be done each year. Don't be as ambitious with the shears as you were with the apple trees.

Often trees produce too much fruit. I don't worry about cherry trees. Let them produce as many cherries as possible. Plums, apples, and peaches must be thinned if the set is overly heavy. I go through and knock off the small, spotted, wormy, and bad fruit when it is about one-third grown. By so doing, the remainder matures in much better shape. At times this thinning process may call for knocking down half of the premature crop or more.

"Where the Apple Reddens"

A large, fruit-covered apple tree became the source of quite a bit of excitement while I was living in Africa. This true account illustrates how easily things can get out of hand when food becomes scarce.

We were in the Congo shortly after the second upheaval, living in the deserted compound of a departed missionary. Apparently the old boy had been there a number of years running a leper colony. Not too many months earlier, the rebels had come through and stripped out all of the plumbing used for the water baths to treat the lepers. They converted the tubs and pipes into stills and made beer and a crude kind of liquor. The followers of the old gent were powerless to preserve the facilities they knew were their only means of survival.

Shortly after we moved in, we noticed a rugged old apple tree growing in the back courtyard. Our understanding was that the old missionary brought the tree from America when he came to the

Congo fifty years earlier. After a time it flowered and set fruit. By the end of the second month the people were already pestering us for the little green apples.

Time went by. The apples matured and the persistent requests continued. Every native, it seemed, wanted to chow down on those apples.

One night we got word that terrorists were going to hit our compound. The warning came in sufficient time for us to be reasonably prepared. A heck of a donnybrook ensued, lasting off and on for about two hours. At dawn the shooting subsided. Shortly thereafter the terrorists withdrew. From the looks of the area, they had sustained some casualties, but managed to evacuate them.

Incredible as it sounds, the object of the terrorist raid was that damn apple tree. These guys were apparently so hungry they tried to shoot their way in to capture our apples!

I pray that things never get that bad in the good old U.S. of A.

Berries

Readers should at least give some thought to raising berries. In some areas, certain kinds of berries do very well, and can be gathered in such a way that they provide a net gain in calories.

Wild berries, by and large, are not practical. Huckleberries, for instance, can be extremely abundant some years. Still, one has to drive to the country to get to them and then it will take two hours or more to collect a gallon. They are okay to make syrup or to season pancakes and rolls, but it's not practical to live on them.

Usually strawberries are not practical. Wild ones are very small. Tame ones require a lot of work. Most varieties have to be replanted every third year.

There are areas where currants and gooseberries grow okay. This tends to be a local phenomenon. Survivalists can't count on them unless past experience indicates otherwise.

About the only berry I know of that comes anywhere near to meeting my practical criteria are raspberries or their close cousins, marion berries, blackberries, and boysenberries. Even these require good solid nursery stock to start with and constant care thereafter.

At present we have twenty-two raspberry bushes growing in our garden. We started with six canes that we soaked in water and stuck in the ground. All grew and sent out runners. We chopped out any starts closer than 3 feet to the parent. Today we have a widely-spaced plot that yields about ten gallons of berries a year.

Each fall the old canes have to be cut out. The new shoots are tied to a stake and in spring cut back severely.

Readers should study their own areas carefully before jumping into the berry business. It generally isn't all that worthwhile.

13. Tanning Skins the Indian Way

If you are *not* a regular hunter or outdoorsman, you have a definite advantage when it comes to home-tanning skins. You won't be predisposed to think the process is too difficult to undertake with rudimentary tools, and will look at every skin that comes into your possession as being something of potential value, which it definitely is.

Too many outdoorsmen shoot cats or groundhogs and never think about saving the skin. Cat skins are tough and durable. They make excellent quality work gloves. Most hunters just bang cats in the head to stop the depredation of native wildlife. Groundhogs have hair, rather than fur. The pelt is not a desirable one in most people's eyes. Yet some of the finest, softest, and most durable leather around can be made from groundhog hides.

Other good examples are rabbit and squirrel skins, and deer hides. All are excellent sources of tanning material that woodsmen tend to throw away. Millions of pounds of these skins are left to rot every year.

As I have said so many times in this book, whatever we do in terms of survival has to provide a net gain in energy. That's why I feel it is futile to make cloth, weave rugs, or indulge in similar macrame-type projects while trying to survive.

Manufacturing furs and leather is different, though. After one gets on to it, the process is relatively easy and not particularly time consuming. The end results are items such as warm blankets, waterproof pants, gloves, hats, rain slickers, and boots. All of these will have to be replaced as they wear out in a long-term survival situation, anyway.

Tanning hides is conveniently divided into several categories. Skins with fur are made into fur, and used principally to stay warm. Hides that are hair covered are made into leather.

In my mind, there are two basic types of leather: buckskin and regular leather. Using mechanical techniques, heavy hides from horses or cattle can be polished down or split to make just about any weight leather desired. But as a practical matter, the survivalist should plan on using the skin as it came from the critter. Forget about splitting or planing pelts. Rather than trying to plane down elk skins, for example, use the leather only for boots, shoes, harnesses, and straps. Softer, thinner goat skin not suited for footwear makes fine raw material for shirts, and so on.

Tanning Supplies

Home tanning does not require a large inventory of equipment. There are only a few materials and tools needed to do an excellent job. Yet trying to get along without this minimum list is the pits. It virtually can't be done.

The first, most important item the prospective tanner is going to need is water. Lots and lots of pure, cool, clean water that has not been chlorinated and does not contain fluoride, and that is *not* hard. Water pumped from a well that contains iron or calcium will not work. Some stream and/or lake water also is impossible to use in the tanning process. It contains too many dissolved minerals and organic pollutants.

A quick rule-of-thumb method to determine if the water you have is fit for tanning use is to wash your hands in it. It is best to use homemade lye soap, although any soap will do. If there is a scum, ring, or layer in the pan when you're done, that water won't work to tan hides.

When we were kids, Dad soaked the hides he tanned in large wooden barrels that originally held dried buttermilk. Several times he made wooden containers by cutting a large five-foot oak log in half and hollowing out the inside with hot rocks and a chisel.

Nowadays I use plastic garbage pails. Anything inert that won't be corroded away by the chemicals is fine. I like plastic because of its light weight and because the containers can be completely cleaned. We had to use old wooden barrels for just one type of soaking mixture. Being able to switch is much more convenient.

Another piece of equipment you will need is a fleshing beam. They are not hard to make, just time consuming. I use an 18-inch hardwood log that is 8 to 10 feet long. Legs or a support structure

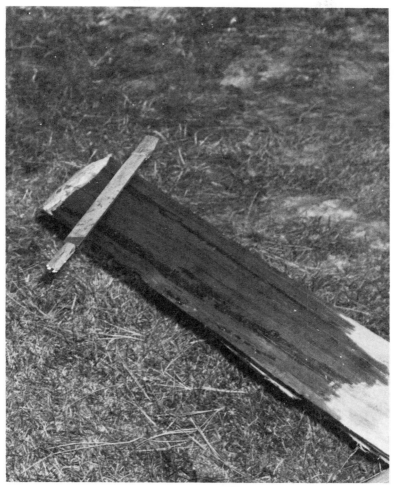

A fleshing beam with scraper made from an old draw file. One end of the fleshing beam is anchored firmly on the ground, with the other working end placed over a log support. The top and working end of the beam must be rounded and smoothed to prevent skins from tearing while they are being worked on.

must be provided that hold the log at a convenient working height. Bevel the end of the beam down, remove the bark, and smooth away all of the knots, branch stubs, and rough spots. This step is very important. You will have a devil of a time keeping holes from being torn in the skins if the beam is rough.

The last item needed is a scraper. It is possible to use a dull single-bladed ax or an old file. I like to make something with handles, much like an old-fashioned spoke shaver. An old piece of 1-inch angle iron works beautifully.

Tanning, as much as is possible, should be done in summer when it is warm. The chemical process goes on much faster, and one can spread out, messing up the backyard rather than the house.

Dermestid beetles will ruin fall- and winter-caught skins by the following summer if special precautions are not taken. Under survival conditions, those special precautions will probably be starting the tanning process. Even heavy salting is of no real help. The beetles eat the skins anyway after it gets warm.

Stretching and Drying

How the skins are initially stretched and dried, before tanning, is important. Fur-type skins are put on premade stretchers of the correct size. No salt is used on small game skins.

Deerskins are spread flat on the floor, flesh side up, and covered with an eighth-inch layer of fine salt. Be sure to flatten down any curling edges before salting. Handle moose, antelope, elk, and caribou skins the same way.

Groundhog-type animals that will be used for leather should be skinned flat and tacked to a board to dry. A little salt can be used if necessary.

Bearskins are greasy, tough buggers to dry thoroughly. The best method is to put them on a slightly sloping floor and salt heavily. After the liquids run off for a day or so, salt again and fold into a square bundle, about 30 inches square. Keep as much salt in the package as possible. Tie together with a piece of rope. Cattle, sheep, and goat skins should also be salted, drained, and bundled for storage. Sometimes I have had as many as eight or ten sitting in the corner of my barn waiting to be tanned.

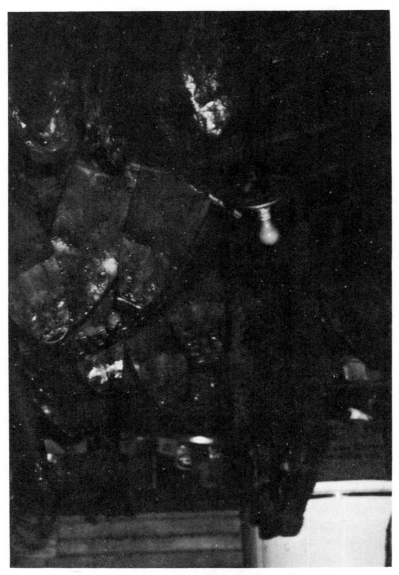

Hanging at left are a bunch of muskrat pelts on stretchers, all caught in snares or a barrel trap. At right is a drying bobcat skin taken in a rabbit snare. All skins must be dried properly before the tanning process can begin.

All skins, great and small, must be skinned clean and fleshed properly before stretching and drying. I can't emphasize this too much. Leave the fat and chunks of meat on the carcass, not on the skin.

The Tanning Process

Some of the following tanning steps apply to one kind of skin and not others. In many cases, not all the processes will be needed. Also, keep in mind that skins wear poorly if they are overtanned. Be sure you sort out which steps are important, and which do not apply to the type of skins you are processing.

Tanning skins is not particularly difficult, although the results come more quickly and easily after a few trial runs. The principal problem is all of the hard, dirty handwork that is sometimes required.

I have listed all the possible steps. Again, be sure they apply to the skins you are treating.

The first step applies to all leather, fur, and buckskin. Pour sufficient clean, soft water—rainwater will do if nothing else is available—in a barrel to cover the skins. Be very cautious if the hide is bone-dry and must be folded to fit in the barrel. It might break. You may have to sprinkle the skins with water to soften them before they can be stuffed into this soaking barrel.

Soak the skins till they are wet through and through. This takes from four hours to five days in the case of big, thick cowhides.

After the hide is thoroughly soaked, take it out of the water, wring it out and flesh it on the beam. Remove all of the remaining fat and grease. Go over the hide and break down the fibers on the flesh side of the skin. On thin, furry skins such as muskrats and mink, the scraping tool is dragged over the skin lightly. On heavy elk hides, hunker down and give it a good scraping. The skin should come out clean and free of blood, dirt, loose hair, grease, and flesh.

Hides that are destined to become leather are placed in a soup made of either 1½ pounds of unslaked lime per 10 gallons of water, or a full 1-gallon pail of hardwood ashes mixed with every 20 gallons of water. Again, use pure water. Mix the solution slowly beforehand, and let it sit for at least two days before putting the skins in it. This lime soaking process loosens the hair on the skins. It is used only when the end result is to be leather.

Unslaked lime can be made by taking regular limestone or sea-shells and heating them thoroughly over a fire. The product must be well burnt and then ground into as fine a powder as possible.

After from two to eight days, depending on the temperature and thickness of the skin, the hair will loosen. Loosening, in this case, means that the hair can be rubbed off the skin easily with a scraper or even the heel of one's hand.

At this point the hide is taken from the lime or ash solution, and the hair along with a bit of the skin layer below it are scraped away. Do this on the fleshing beam. Small, light skins require a light going over. Heavy cow or horse hides should be scraped with vigor.

Some thinning of the hides can be done at this time. As I said previously, it is folly for home tanners to attempt to shave down entire skins, but they can polish down a few very thick spots over the shoulders and on the neck.

The lime dehairing process works faster and in a more even fashion when the solution is stirred often. I use an old canoe paddle to give it a few whirls each day.

Place the freshly scraped hides in a barrel of clean water to soak. The old lime water is good for the garden, if it becomes necessary to dump it. Soak for twenty-four hours, remove, and wring out.

Dump out the water, and fill the barrel again with clean water. Add 1 gallon of vinegar or 3 gallons of sour milk and soak the skins again. Calf or groundhog skins should soak for about eight hours. Heavier skins need about a day.

Remove the skins, and rinse in fresh water. They are now ready for tanning. If you are making skins with fur on them, the following is the first step after the initial soak and scraping process.

This method is a fine, relatively easy way of tanning leather or fur that makes use of naturally occurring, easily obtained materials. In times past when chemicals such as alum or sulfuric acid were not available, it was all there was. Today the process is not used because it is so slow. Warm weather speeds things up, but still we are talking four weeks for small, thin furs such as mink, and up to five months for thick elk or moose hides.

Historically the technique has been known as *bark tanning*. It makes use of tannic acid salvaged from oak bark, sumac leaves,

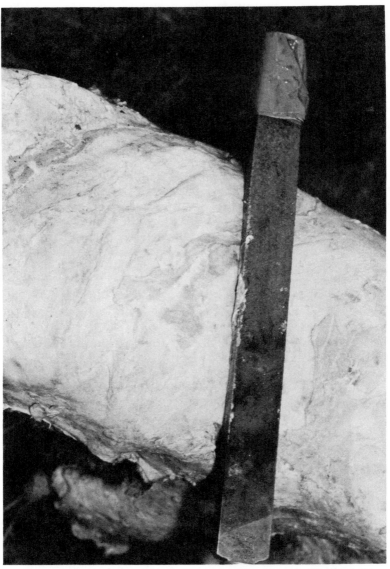

After the skin has been initially soaked in clean water, it is placed on the fleshing beam. Use the scraper to remove all excess flesh and fat from the skin. This step also breaks down the structure on the hide itself, ensuring a better tan.

buckeye bark and nuts, or other similar materials. Some old-timers like myself don't like to use bark on furs because of the staining effect. This does not, however, preclude using natural materials. There is always the tannic acid extract from ground, leached acorns. The extract works much faster and better than straight bark, and will not dye the hides as dark as the other method.

For each gallon of acorn leaching, add 2 gallons of good clean soft water. The original liquid must be good and sour, leached from finely ground acorn meal. Prepare enough liquid to totally submerge the hide. If acorn juice is not available, fine-grind oak or sumac bark and pour boiling water over it. Use about 35 pounds of bark for 50 gallons of water.

Let the tanning liquid sit for two weeks, then filter through a cloth and use it as is without further dilution.

Place the barrel with hides someplace warm with convenient access. The hides should be stirred at least twice a day. If you have it, a half-gallon of vinegar per 50 gallons of water will speed the process.

Change the mixture every thirty days till the tanning process is completed. You can tell when this has happened by cutting a thin slice out of the thickest section of the hide. Usually this is the neck. A very thin, light brown line should be visible coming in from each side of the hide or fur. Tanning is completed when the lines converge and no light or white-colored streak remains in the center of the skin.

Rabbit skins take four weeks minimum. Elk or moose leather destined to become belts, straps, or shoe soles will take three months minimum. Very heavy hides should be left at least thirty days longer after it seems they have tanned all the way through.

After tanning is completed, the hide can be colored by soaking it in walnut hulls and water for a few days. Another method is to hang the skin over a smoky, punky fire and leave it for a day or two. Some methods of tanning produce ghostly white skins that have to be colored, they look so bad. This is not entirely true with bark tanning, but you will have to be the judge of this.

After tanning, the hide fibers must be broken so that they will remain soft. As the hide dries, it must be pulled and stretched over the fleshing beam. This aspect of the process takes lots of work and

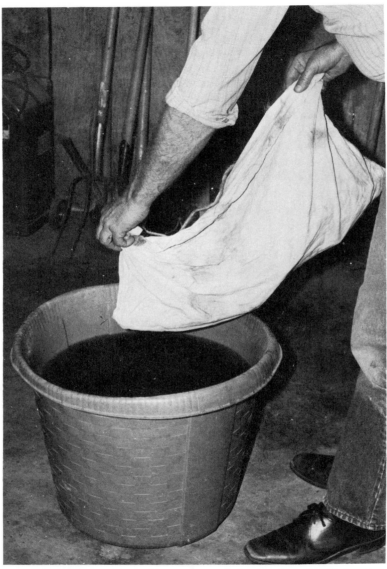

Hair must be removed from skins used to make leather. Lime is added to clean water, and the skins soaked again until the hair comes loose. Hair is then scraped off before continuing the leather-making process.

patience. Little skins break up nicely. Heavy leather requires some work with the scraper.

After the skin is two-thirds dry, begin to oil it lightly as you work it over the beam.

My rule of thumb is to use light animal oils on light skins and heavier oils on thick leather hides. If you have it, rendered duck fat works very well on rabbit or muskrat skins, and possum, coyote, bear, or pork fat is good on elk skins. Don't soak the skin with oil. Apply only as much as the skin will readily absorb.

Making Indian Buckskin

Indian buckskin is made by soaking and scraping the hide, and then soaking it again to loosen the hair. Lime is not used. Plain water will work on buckskin if left for four to five days.

After the hair is scraped, place the hide in a solution of about 2 pounds of homemade soap in 10 gallons of water. Leave for a week and change the solution.

At the end of two weeks, take the skins out and begin working over the beam. As they dry, apply light coats of bear, raccoon, or pork grease. *Mucho* hard labor is required to soften one of these buckskins.

Brain Tanning

Furs can be tanned by boiling the brains of a fairly good-sized animal—a deer brain does a coyote nicely—and applying the paste to the skin. Roll the skin up for one to three days. Wash it off and then begin the softening process. Be sure the skin does not spoil while rolled up with the brain paste. Although widely alluded to in literature that treats the subject lightly, this method is not a particularly good one. It really works only on small, light furs.

After you learn the process, tanning is best done in batches. As a practical matter, it only works in summer.

Before starting, you should have a good idea what you are going to do with the skins. Don't go to all the work required unless you know you will need three deer for shirts, an elk for boot and strap material, groundhogs for hats, cat skins for gloves, and so on.

Don't forget that home-tanned leather and fur can be quite warm and waterproof. Muskrat skins sewn fur-in, backed by goat or calf

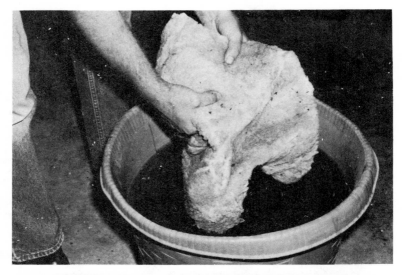

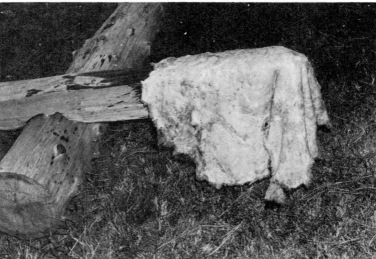

Top: Prepared skins going into final tanning solution made from acorn leachant or bark with heavy tannic acid concentration.

Bottom: After soaking in the tanning solution, the skin is removed and worked over the fleshing beam as it dries. Some neatsfoot oil should be applied as the skin structure is broken down, or native animal fat can be used.

skins that are well oiled, make a rugged, all-weather jacket that will last for years.

Generally we will have clothes around that can be scrounged. The problem may occur when we look for a new pair of shoelaces, some straps, or a new pair of soles for boots. Then it will be nice to know how to use the materials at hand to produce leather and fur.

14. Preserving Food

This is the chapter where we are finally going to lose the purists. After reviewing many, many accurate and obscure methods of preserving food, I am going to make my recommendations. And my advice is going to so upset the "survival for the sake of survival" nut that he might give up right here.

But don't you forget the acid tests for true survival. If it takes more calories to do than are returned in the process, it isn't worth the effort.

Before the 1790s, there was only one set of preservative methods that the world had to work with. Within that set there existed a number of tricks that one could use. The following is a short summary of those old-time tricks and methods.

Uncle's Riddle

One day when I was a lad, Uncle asked me a riddle of sorts. "A fair emergency method of preserving meat," he said, "is to boil it. How do you suppose the Indians boiled water?"

Certainly a good question. Without metal containers it is difficult to pull off this otherwise simple feat. I knew from past conversations with my uncle that Indians often used the boiling method. But for the life of me I couldn't figure out how without a metal pot.

Birch bark cooking utensils were common with the Redman. So were wooden bowls made of cedar or oak. Gourds were another widely used container, but the most interesting were those made from animal parts. Turtle shell bowls with clamshell spoons are some of the more exotic. Raw deer hides, the pouch or stomach, intestines, and the thorax were also used. Clay pots used by some Indians are not a good answer. They transfer heat poorly and will shatter over a hot fire.

The not-so-obvious answer to the riddle is that the Indians pulled hot stones out of their fires and dropped them in their otherwise flammable or breakable containers. They exchanged the hot rocks until the water boiled.

There will probably always be some sort of metal container around for the survivalist to use. But who knows? Some morning you may have to bathe with nothing more than icy stream water in a plastic dishpan. Hot rocks may save the day.

Fairly well boiled meat will last about three days under even the worst of conditions found in the United States. In most cases it will last much longer. Boiling meat is not a viable method of preparing food for extended storage.

Hanging

If the weather is cool, and the game can be protected from flies, either with its natural skin or with a cloth net, it may be preserved for a surprising amount of time by simple hanging.

The secret is to dress the game quickly, leaving the skin or feathers intact. As soon as this is done, hang it up where the air can circulate around it, shaded from as much light as possible. Grouse, pheasants, quail, squirrels, rabbits, and even deer will keep fairly well using this method. Raccoons, possums, and bears are too greasy. Hanging fish won't work at all except for fertilizer.

During warm weather there are two additional measures that will help preserve hanging meat, useful if the reader has the needed materials. Washing the skinned, exposed areas with a 50:50 vinegar-water solution will help keep the flies off. Covering with a piece of cheesecloth also helps.

Meat that can be stored at 55 degrees Fahrenheit or lower can be skinned, covered, and kept very nicely. Often this is how deer or elk are kept in an early fall hunting camp.

Any animals, wild or domestic, become rank after hanging but be assured they *are* edible. My favorite recollection of this method involves a true, personal experience.

I was hare hunting in Scotland and managed to bag three. As per my friend's instruction, I gutted and hung the bunnies from a post stuck in a rock pile fence about sixty yards behind the barn. That night, I left for London and from there flew on to Lisbon, Portugal. Several weeks later I received a card from the woman in whose house I had stayed, scolding me for giving the rabbits to someone else. In due time I wrote back explaining that the meat was probably rotted on the pole in the rock pile where I left it.

When I got back to the States, a letter from my hostess mentioned finding the rabbits. She said they were good eating but chided me for not telling her where they were before I'd left!

Under the most adverse conditions, hung meat will last but three or four days. In much of the U.S., though, it can be kept for from one to as long as five months, depending on the ambient temperature.

Earth Oven Baking

Consider this as much a way of preparing food as of preserving it. Earthen ovens are nothing more than luau-type pits dug in the ground and filled with glowing coals. Edible items can be wrapped in leaves, rawhide, or tinfoil, or placed in metal containers snuggled in the charcoal. Up to a foot of earth is placed over the coals to contain them. Cooked meat and vegetables will last three days at a minimum.

Two favorite techniques come to mind. If a covered metal or clay pot is available, put into it a measure of dried beans together with four measures of water, and a piece of salt meat. Scoop a half-bushel of glowing coals into a large hole, throw in a few rocks, then the pot, and cover the whole works with dirt. Do this before leaving in the morning. By night the mixture will be delicious.

Everyone knows that potatoes can be buried and cooked with coals, but how many know the old Indian trick for baking fresh corn? Pick but don't husk the corn. Soak it in water for thirty minutes and then roast for about forty minutes in an earthen oven.

Leaching

I alluded to this method in the chapter on Indians. You may remember that the native Americans often took unpalatable or poisonous food products, such as acorns, and dissolved off the harmful substances.

Doing this does not require modern containers, but it does help mightily to have some on hand. Before pots, the Indians would leach their acorn meal in a shallow hole dug in a gravel bar along the river. They carefully selected a place where the sand acted as a filter for the water passing through the food.

Let's hope none of us ever becomes that desperate.

The usual process is to coarse-grind the acorn kernels, put them in a pot, and cover with water. Stir a couple of times in the next two hours and then drain off the liquid.

Repeat as many times as needed to remove the offending acids. The survivor can test the goodness of his meal by sampling the water. If it tastes sweet after washing, the acids have been washed away.

Some nuts have more acid than others. There is no hard and fast rule regarding the number of washings that will be required.

Preserve the resulting mixture by drying it thoroughly. Pack the meal into an airtight container. If containers are not available, the meal may be baked into bread or cakes. With but a minimal amount of protection—I put my acorn biscuits in a burlap bag— they will last for at least two years. Taste is not bad, but they sure can get tiresome if that's all there is to eat.

Drying

Apparently the oldest, and most certain primitive method of preserving meat is to dry it. In some climates in our country it is necessary to use artificial heat. This can be the energy from a burning log—not that artificial in my opinion, but different from simply hanging the meat out to dry in the sun.

African bush natives I worked with when I was on the Dark Continent, made a product they called *biltong*. It was identical to our jerky, except for the size of the chunks of meat. The natives commonly dried ten- or twelve- pound kudu shoulders, often leaving the bone in till the process was completed.

In our climate, I find it best to cut the meat into strips no thicker than ½ inch. It isn't necessary if one dries his meat quickly over a fire, but I also soak the strips in a weak salt solution. One cup of salt per gallon of water is close enough. Soak for six hours and remove from the solution. Dry in the sun slightly till the meat is plastic in texture. Lightly rub in a small amount of finely ground pepper. Dry the resulting combination thoroughly. A cheesecloth enclosure will keep flies and bugs off the drying meat.

Drying can be a chore. Wet, cold, or muggy climates are not conducive to it. Midwestern summers, especially, are impossible.

It is better to keep the food on the hoof if possible, till it stands a better chance of drying before going putrid.

Jerky

Wood stoves, fireplaces, a coal-fired reflector oven, or an open campfire can be used to make jerky. Place ½-inch strips of meat on a rack above low, even heat for twelve hours or so. The result should be black, shriveled, hard strips that bite, bend, and chew like greasy leather. The salt and pepper make the product a bit more palatable.

I have never determined the life expectancy of jerky. Given a minimal amount of protection, kept dry and away from the squirrels, it has lasted me eighteen months or more. Under most conditions it should be prepared in fall. If one has a moose on the grass in July, it won't do to wait two months. A fire must be built, racks constructed, and the meat cured now.

Drying Grains, Nuts, and Vegetables

Most vegetables, nuts, or grains should be allowed to dry naturally, if at all possible. Field corn and wheat are wonderful food sources that keep well this way. Leave it in the field till the moisture content drops below 12 percent. Bite the kernel of grain to determine this. If it breaks with a pop, without bending or mashing, it is at or near the proper level.

Nuts are gathered in the fall. Usually they must be spread out and air-dried in an attic or loft. Laying them out in the sun helps, if they won't get rained on or filched by the squirrels.

Acorns, as previously mentioned, must be leached. Walnuts are available in some places in quantity, but may be a poor food source. Most are as bitter as acorns so must be similarly leached. The double hulls are more of a problem though. They take a surprising amount of time to crack out.

Sometimes vegetables can be dried. Corn left on the cob is a good example. In some climates, it will mold before it dries. If that happens, make a rack, start a fire, and get it dried out.

Fish

Fish can be dehydrated for use later. Fatter, greasier fish work best but all can be dried. Little fish in the bluegill class should be cleaned and scaled lightly. Place them whole on a rack over a fire that will produce a generous amount of heat. Fish need to be dried with haste or they spoil.

Larger fish must be split lengthwise and the halves placed on racks to dry. Salmon, trout, sturgeon, and steelhead dry very nicely. Pike, walleye, and perch have larger scales and don't seem to dry as well. Carp will dry, but there are better ways to keep these over-grown goldfish.

Tiny-boned fish, such as suckers, whitefish, and mooneyes, can be dried. Under most circumstances the result is very palatable. Again, there are better ways to handle these guys.

Dried fish is quite nutritious and very filling. It will store quite well. Generally, I dry fish for dog feed, when I have lots of them (both dogs and fish).

A fish-drying rack can be made of metal or wood. Two old sets of bedsprings are ideal. Tie the rack together at the top and set them up so they lean together at a 35-degree angle. Tie the fish on the racks a row at a time, using grass, wire, or branches.

Build a fire inside the bedsprings and keep it going till the fish dehydrate. Generally this takes about two days.

Drying Fruits

Some fruits should be dried. Some keep well if stored correctly but peaches, pears, grapes, and plums all must be dried. Cherries do not dry well and apples can go either way.

I recommend that apples be stored, if possible, and then dried in the winter when the heat will also warm the house.

For drying, fruit should be sliced about ⅜-inch thick, cored or pitted but not peeled, and placed on a rack that will allow the warm air to circulate up from the bottom. In some climates, supplemental heat will be required.

I use a piece of ¼-inch hardware cloth for the racks, or in the case of grapes, a piece of screen. Plums are usually best left with the pits in.

Be sure the heat is mild and as consistent as possible. Lots of low-humidity air should pass through the fruit.

Consistent slicing helps immensely. Otherwise, the thin pieces will dry first and must be laboriously picked out of the batch. Don't

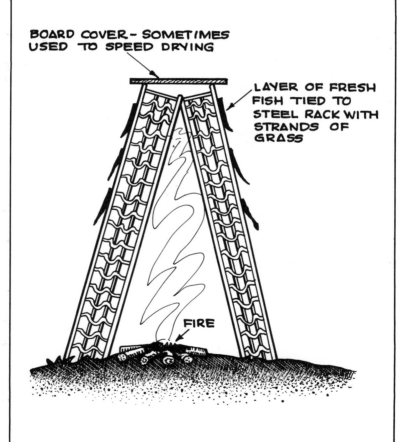

DRYING OR SMOKING RACK
MADE FROM BEDSPRINGS

BOARD COVER – SOMETIMES
USED TO SPEED DRYING

LAYER OF FRESH
FISH TIED TO
STEEL RACK WITH
STRANDS OF
GRASS

FIRE

try to dry dissimilar types of fruit together. Sliced apples and plums, for example, won't dehydrate well in the same rack.

Dried fruit keeps quite well, but not forever. I generally try to turn my fall supply to calories by the next spring.

Fruit Leather

Bushels and bushels of fruit can be stored as fruit leather if you have no other means of storage and also have a great surplus of raw fruit.

We make our fruit leather mostly out of plums. Sometimes they turn out pretty sour so we add a little sugar. Generally all it takes is lots of plums, pears, cherries, apples, peaches, and pears. Some of the best leather is made from two or three fruits mixed together.

Presently it is common for folks to make small batches of the stuff using a blender. The best way I know of is to run a bushel of fruit through a big meat grinder a couple of times. Although it isn't absolutely necessary, it is best to take the cores out of apples and pears. Peaches, plums, and cherries have to be pitted. If you want to fool with it, filter the liquid away from the apples to use in making vinegar.

Spread the soup made from the fruit out about ⅜-inch deep on cookie sheets and dry in the oven or in the sun till the residue has the consistency of soft rubber. Lift the dried sheets of fruit leather with a spatula, roll into tubes, cut and put in wide-mouthed jars.

Fruit leather will keep at least six months this way. It is very good tasting, besides being a real treat in the middle of the winter when the frost is on the pumpkin.

Berries in Lard

Berries are difficult to store using primitive methods. They dehydrate to nothing and spoil quickly under most other normal circumstances. I always get a laugh out of people who ask me if I can live on berries in the woods. Obviously they have never tried to live off the land in the woods.

Wild berries require a lot of energy to pick. There usually are not enough to actually live on, and what berries do appear are seasonal. They might last a week or ten days and then are gone for another year.

One primitive method of keeping berries is to seal them in a container with lard. Coon and bear fat, pork lard, deer tallow, or beef fat can all be used. A tin can, skin pouch, cleaned intestine, metal bucket, birch bark container, or anything similar works adequately for the container.

Pack the berries in the receptacle and pour the melted grease in around the berries, making a solid mass. The resulting package keeps fairly well, carries nicely, and makes for the best heartburn since eating live toads.

Rendering Lard

Perhaps most folks who read this book know how to render fat into lard. Lard can come in handy, so a short explanation follows.

Wild and domestic animals sometimes have a large quantity of fat built up in their bodies. The material has a great number of uses for everything from cooking, to preserving food, to making boot waterproofing. The problem is preserving it.

Start by stripping the raw fat out of the animal. Cut it away from the skin and the outside of the carcass, and collect it from inside the body cavity.

Put all of the fat in a heavy metal container and heat. Lard from various animals should be rendered separately, especially bear from deer, or hog from cattle.

The mixture will bubble furiously as the heat drives off the water and melts down the fat. Large batches work best, so do as much as possible in the biggest kettle available. After a bit, the chunks will melt down, and just about stop bubbling.

Pour the lard into a can where it will be stored and if possible, squeeze the pieces left in the pot. Elaborate lard presses have been made for this use but may not be available.

Residue pieces are called *cracklins*. People eat them but my pooches enjoy them more.

Grinding

Grinding can be used to preserve a meat-based material called *pemmican*. The method yields a food that literally will keep for years, and also is pretty good tasting. The work that is involved putting it up can be considerable, though.

Other than the same old skin, bark, wooden, metal, or plastic containers that are always required, you will need equal parts of melted fat, jerky, and berries or other fruit. Usually when I make pemmican, I save the tallow from my winter deer. As soon as the blackberries or huckleberries are on in summer, I start the pemmican process.

Take the dried meat you have selected and grind or pound it into pulp. The finer the better. Melt the lard, and mash the berries well. Mix the whole thing together in equal parts and pour into containers. I use rolled tubes made of three layers of freezer paper.

Pemmican provides a good means of storing valuable foods, but is a bit cumbersome to prepare.

Smoking Meat

I smoke all my meat in a simple covered barbecue. Some folks build smokers out of old refrigerators or even make smokehouses out of logs. Out in the bush, I build smoking racks similar to those used to dry fish, usually from green limbs and wire I bring along.

The basic plan when smoking any meat or vegetable is to keep the fire as cool as possible and as smokey as practical, by feeding in wet or green logs, or throwing a few scoops of dirt on the blaze.

For all-around use at home or retreat, a barbecue with a tight lid is definitely the best bet. I stoke mine with apple wood, opening the air vent just enough to let the chips smolder.

Smoked meat keeps reasonably well, and tastes a whole lot better than meat preserved by other methods. The harder and cooler the product is smoked, the longer it will last in storage.

Greasy meats smoke best. Pork, bear, coons, ducks, and geese are a few examples.

In fall when the ducks are still very fat, I smoke every one I can get. Start by dissolving about 1½ pounds of salt in 4 to 5 gallons of water. Soak the ducks for twenty-four hours if they are large ones with good body fat. Smaller ducks can be soaked well enough in eighteen hours.

Build a small chip fire in the barbecuer. Dry the ducks and put as many as will fit on the top rack inside. It will take about eight hours to thoroughly smoke them. During that time, the fire will have to be maintained to keep it from going out or from running out of fuel. Try to make as smokey a fire as possible with as little heat as possible.

Excess heat is not near the problem it is with an open fire. The grabber in open fire conditions is the large amount of fuel that must be consumed to get the job done outdoors, and the fact that it takes two to three days.

Elk, deer, moose, and beef are not particularly good smoked. At least I don't think they are. However, they can be preserved in a sort of black, chewy, tough form.

Smoking is an excellent method of preparing and preserving fish. The method works especially well for greasy, bony fish that normally aren't particularly tasty. Carp, bullheads, suckers, redhorses, whitefish, gar, and similar protein sources are good examples. Other more desirable fish in the salmon, pike, walleye, bass class are even better when smoked.

Dissolve 1½ pounds of salt in 4 gallons of water and soak the fish five hours. More salt is fine if you like saltier fish. Split the larger fish—over 2½ pounds—in half but do not scale any of them. Dry the fish and place on the smoke rack or barbecue grill skin side toward the smoke. It takes about four hours to cure them.

Raccoons and possums are very good smoked. Rabbits and squirrels dry out too much. Use 2 pounds of salt to 4 gallons of water, twenty-four hours to smoke and about twelve hours to do small three- to eight-pound animals.

Some vegetables are good smoked. The Nez Perce Indians cured camas roots over a smoky fire. The resulting product kept a minimum of one year and was really quite good. Smoked camas tastes like a fire-cured potato with the texture of an onion.

Salting

Any meat and some vegetables—cucumbers and cabbage—can be preserved for a few years in a salt brine.

The procedure is relatively simple but the end product is not terribly nutritious. When used after storage, the salt must be removed from the food with repeated washings of cool, clean water. At a place where fresh water is at a premium, this can be a problem.

I bone all meat I intend to salt-cure and cut into pieces weighing not over four pounds. Fish must be gutted and if large, split in half. Chickens, squirrels, and rabbits can be salt-cured whole. Turkeys, geese, and large ducks must be split in half.

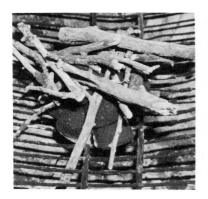
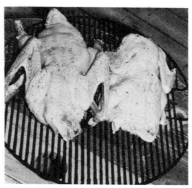
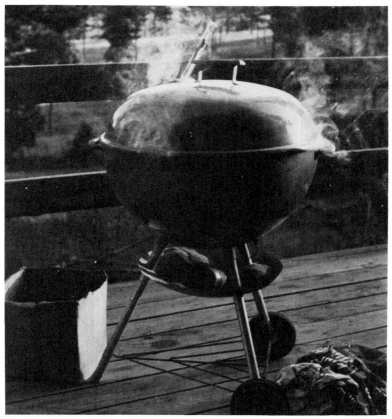

Smoking ducks with a standard, enclosed barbecue grill. (*1*) Briquets and apple wood twigs at bottom of grill, ready to light. (*2*) Ducks after soaking in salt water, ready for smoking. (*3*) Grill during smoking process. Note thermometer stuck in top vent hole. At 140 degrees, smoking takes about five hours.

Roll the meat in salt till it is covered and no more salt will stick. Place in a wood or plastic container and allow to sit for twenty-four hours. Pour off the liquid and submerge in a salt brine concentrated enough to float a potato.

Be sure to use a noncorrosive container to store your salted supplies in. A plastic restaurant bucket with lid is ideal.

Cabbage, cucumbers, and corn can be preserved in a similar solution. Eating this stuff makes survival a borderline deal. It will keep three or four years.

Root Cellars

A root cellar is simply a buried room with a door. Being underground, the temperature stays even at about 60 degrees Fahrenheit and the humidity remains constant, going neither very high nor very low.

Good solid root cellars are built out of concrete with a paved walk and stairs leading to the door. The last one I built had concrete walls, an earth floor, wooden shelves, and was lined and roofed with a double layer of corrugated tin roofing. It was about 6 feet square, had two roof supports, and an old wooden door from an abandoned farmhouse. We could store more than enough food in it to last the winter for our family of five. At one time the temperature reached 22 degrees below zero. According to our little thermometer inside the door, the temperature in the root cellar never went below 55 degrees Fahrenheit. The three feet of soil on the roof provided excellent insulation.

Root cellars cannot, as a general rule, be built in the basements of houses. They end up being insulated poorly. The temperature and humidity fluctuate and the produce spoils.

Instead, locate your root cellar on a high, dry, well-drained piece of ground not subject to water seepage. Make sure the roof is watertight and the door seals well. A small ceiling vent must be run through the top dirt to the outside. I make mine out of 2-inch plastic pipe with a bug screen and tin can hat to keep out the varmints and the rain.

Root cellars can be used as fallout shelters.

Ice House

For those who have access to quantities of winter ice, piles of sawdust, good logs for construction, cutting tools, and a way to

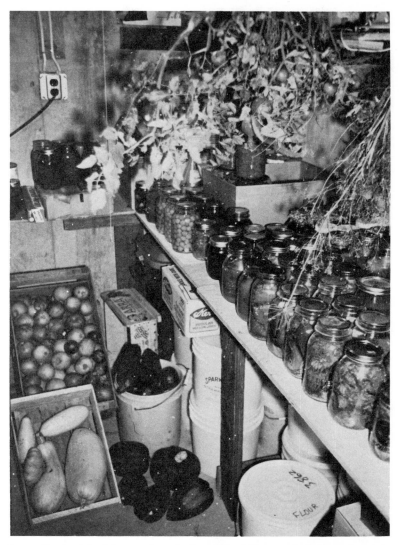

Root cellar loaded with canned goods, dry edibles in restaurant buckets, ripening fruit and vegetables, and other supplies. Note tomato vines hanging from ceiling. Cut just before the frost, they will ripen nicely through the winter.

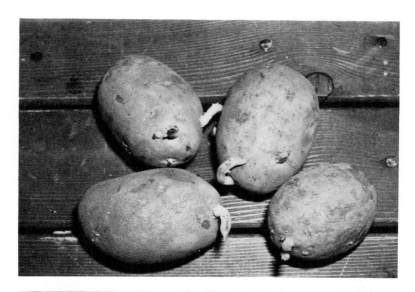

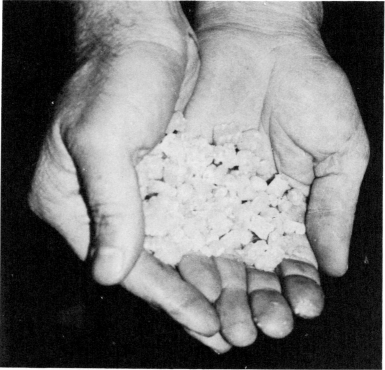

Top: Sprouted potatoes. A root cellar is the best possible place to store spuds. *Bottom:* Dried corn. This grain is easy to grow, easy to dry, and easy to store. The author suggests growing field corn in place of garden varieties.

haul the ice to the storage area, an ice house may be of interest. Most survivalists won't be able to put all this together, but perhaps some will. Maybe I will even be able to trade with you for some of your ice.

For the ice house structure, you will need a very stout log pen. In all cases it should be as high as it is wide—about 14 feet on a side. Logs should be no less than 12 inches in diameter, and well chinked.

Put a raised roof on the pen. The peak of the roof should start about 3 feet above the pen and overhang it no less than 3 feet.

Put blocks of ice 3 feet square on a 1-foot bed of sawdust inside the completed log pen. Stack the ice 6 feet high in 3-foot rows with a foot of space between the rows. Fill all these empty spaces with sawdust, covering the top row of ice with a foot or more. Put in the second ice block layer the same as the first, and so on. Ice packed in sawdust like this will last two years.

Sugar Curing

Game can be preserved by keeping it in a solution of sugar. But in my estimate it is a dumb solution to the problem of storing food.

When the time comes, salt will be a valuable commodity indeed. Sugar will be even more valuable than salt. Egyptians used honey to preserve food but I don't anticipate a surplus of honey, either.

For those who want to experiment, dissolve enough sugar in water to float our proverbial potato and sink the meat. It will keep if completely covered. Meat such as pork, deer, and elk tastes reasonably good cured in sugar. Sugar-cured fish are horrible.

Live Storage

A few years back we ran into a tremendous small mouth bass situation. A new reservoir near us had aged sufficiently so that it started producing these fish in large quantities.

We caught a great many in fish traps and with hook and line. The problem was how to store all the fish.

Eventually we solved the problem by releasing the live bass in a closed pool formed when a side creek overflowed and dug out a hole. The pool was about sixty yards long by approximately eight

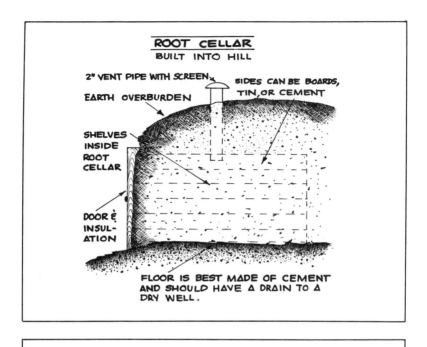

ROOT CELLAR
BUILT INTO HILL

2" VENT PIPE WITH SCREEN

EARTH OVERBURDEN

SIDES CAN BE BOARDS, TIN, OR CEMENT

SHELVES INSIDE ROOT CELLAR

DOOR & INSUL-ATION

FLOOR IS BEST MADE OF CEMENT AND SHOULD HAVE A DRAIN TO A DRY WELL.

END VIEW OF ICE HOUSE
NO END WALL SHOWING

3-FOOT SQUARE BLOCKS OF ICE

ONE-FOOT SAWDUST NEXT TO WALL AND OVER TOP OF FIRST LAYER

ONE-FOOT DEEP LAYER OF SAWDUST TO START ON

yards wide. Some water apparently filtered in and out through the gravel, as it seemed clean and fresh enough.

I don't know how many bass we put in the little pond, but there were quite a few. During the summer we took them out with hook and line, as needed. During the fall some coons started working our fishpond and we trapped three of them as well.

My point is that many wild animals and semiwild animals can be left out alive and well till the time of need. It's generally a much easier system than trying to preserve them for the winter.

Pigeons are a good example. They don't migrate. One can expect to find them in the same roosts month after month. They are somewhat like a bunch of chickens in this sense. Unless there are other factors encountered, I recommend taking a few now and then as needed, and allowing the others to go their merry way.

Turtles, especially snappers, are an outstanding source of food that should be stored alive. Catch them in midsummer. Drill a hole in the edge of the shell and fasten to a root or rock with a piece of number 9 wire. I have kept them this way up to fourteen months, tethered on 12 feet of wire. They seem to get plenty to eat, and even fatten a bit.

My grandparents used to keep catfish in old buttermilk barrels. The catfish also seemed to fatten up a bit before slaughter.

Bullheads are another fish that can be kept alive in any old pond for long periods of time. Often I have emptied my fish traps of them into a little 6-by-6-foot pond. Three months later they are still in excellent shape.

Carp, and even trout, can be penned into small tributaries when the water is high. Within reasonable limits they will still be there later on after the water has gone down and the other fish have all moved downstream.

Some game should not be harvested till needed unless there is a chance that someone else will get it. Clams and oysters don't move terribly far. Leave them in place till immediately before hunger pangs hit.

Keeping wild game in semiconfinement should be viewed in contrast to keeping purely domestic animals. In a pure survival situation it may become practical to keep a few rabbits on the back porch or some goats in the yard. The difference between controlling wild game and keeping domestic animals is responsibility.

Wild critters basically take care of themselves, while their domestic relatives will rely on you for food, shelter, and protection.

Eggs

In a cool environment, eggs can be kept for very long periods of time. We have stored them in our root cellar from September to May, when the chickens started laying again.

Eggs can be kept in a warm climate by covering them with a solution of sodium silicate. This is an old-time product commonly called *water glass*. It is available at most drug stores and is reasonably priced.

The solution should be concentrated enough so that it almost floats a fresh egg. A good test is to move the eggs up and down in the water and water glass solution. They should stabilize at the level they are placed at without rising or sinking.

Canning

Some forgotten Frenchman developed the science of canning meat and vegetables. By so doing he allowed another Frenchman—Napoleon—to march off to war at the head of the first army that no longer had to rely on feeding itself with what it found along its route of march.

I have in my various survival caches a total of about five hundred canning jar lids. As most folks know, canning lids are the Achilles' heel of the home canner. Hoarding them is logical. However, I doubt if we ever will use them. In all likelihood the lids will be used for trading stock.

Home canning is a moderately technical process yielding a reasonably good product under some conditions. Many good manuals are available on the subject. On the other hand, home canning can be dangerous, expensive in terms of human energy, and uncertain.

It is virtually impossible to safely can fish or seafood. Assuming that one is successful having braved botulism and the vagaries of an uncertain product, the end result is so stripped of taste and food value that it is virtually worthless.

Meat and vegetables can be canned in glass jars. Under some circumstances it is even easier than smoking or drying. The catch comes when one tries to can these items using only makeshift equipment.

Most manuals on canning recommend that meat, poultry, and vegetables sterilized in an open water bath be boiled for three to three and a half hours. An increase of thirty minutes per five hundred feet of elevation above sea level must be figured in as well. At the elevation I now live at, using an open kettle, I would have to boil glass jars a minimum of seven hours! To do less would risk spoilage and botulism.

Use of a pressure cooker cuts the time needed back to one or one and a half hours, but still this may not be acceptable. Unless you have access to a good stove there will still be problems. Wood stoves are fine, but an open campfire is not.

Berries and fruit are relatively simple to can. The boiling time is only about thirty minutes in an open container; fruit contains acid which kills botulism. Fruit such as peaches, plums, and cherries are difficult to preserve with some other methods. Canning these makes more sense.

Freezing

When the crash comes, I plan on using a number of different methods to preserve my food. But after giving the whole matter a great deal of thought, I have decided that the best plan available for me is to freeze all of my fish, poultry, and red meat, all of my vegetables that won't keep in the root cellar, and some of the berries and soft fruit.

I am sure that many of the survival purists' hair is standing on end right now, but as I see it, it's a matter of economics. As I have said many times, survival after a collapse is going to be tough. The ones who make it are going to be the ones who are prepared, and will use every means at their disposal. They cannot expend more energy than they store just for the sake of using some neat survival technique they read about in the library one afternoon.

My reasoning here involves nutrition and convenience. The easiest, safest, quickest way to preserve meat and vegetables is in a freezer. One simply wraps the pieces in reusable paper and puts them in the machine. Vegetables must be blanched and cooled, but it's not much work.

My two freezers have 1/6-horsepower motors and consume about 1½ kilowatts of electricity on a hot July day. Even if I load them up it will take less than three days to freeze the load at a cost of about 33 kilowats.

Since I need electrical power to run my water pump anyway, and since I have a beautiful little diesel generator (see chapter 18 for information on generators) that runs on about a half-gallon of fuel a day, I have concluded that the best method of preserving most of our family's food is to freeze it.

My 1,000-gallon underground storage tank has enough oil to generate all the power I need for at least four years. This is assuming I no longer use the fuel as a back-up to heat with and switch entirely to wood.

If after three or four years things have not improved, I can always plan to switch to the other food preservation techniques. When the crash comes, you and I, the ones who make it, are going to have to work our tails off. It will be important to be as efficient as possible. Preserving food by freezing fits into that philosophy.

15. Old-Time Potpourri

One of these days some of us old-timers are going to have to sit down and come up with a list of all the old-fashioned formulas we know. A lot of this knowledge is in danger of passing into permanent oblivion within a few years—just at the time when this country will need it again.

The following chapter is not all-inclusive. I suspect it isn't even logical in some places. It's just a lot of fun to go over some of the old formulas we used to have and tell other people about them. Some of the products are still better than anything that can be purchased in shops today.

The first example is one of the best.

Snowshoe Dressing

Use slightly warmed, rendered duck or goose fat on snowshoe webs. Simple as that. Be sure not to get salt in the dressing, since it is hard on leather.

Pastry Shortening

Bear lard is the best pastry shortening there is. Coon and possum lard come a close second. As with all animal fats, the chunks should be trimmed free of muscle tissue and boiled till they stop bubbling. Smaller pieces render more efficiently.

The residual chunks should be pressed if possible and then cooled for dog food. Oil drained from the rendering pot should be stored in airtight bottles. Label each container so you know what you have in each, and do not mix them. A root cellar is a good place to store this type of product.

Boot Dressing

Boot uppers are best treated with rendered beaver fat, or skunk oil works well. Skunk oil isn't nearly as rank as you might first imagine. Rendering seems to kill a lot of the odor. Beaver oil has a very pleasant smell.

Boot Welt Waterproofing

I like a mixture of lard and beeswax, or tallow and beeswax for treating boot welts. Done correctly, it will waterproof boots better than anything else I have ever used.

Melt the lard and the beeswax over a low flame in a shallow pan. Put the boots in the pan and leave them there a few minutes to soak up the waterproofing. This trick for leather boots should be a military secret.

Eating Utensils

Whether camping, hunting, or whatever outdoors, I use two thin branches as chopsticks. I first learned to use chopsticks to eat with in the Orient. Now I use them all the time when I camp. They are *so* convenient. Readers might keep this in mind. No washing, no mess, no fuss. Throw them in the fire when you are done.

Dye

Red beets make fairly good red dye. Walnut hulls produce a nice brown color. Willow leaves and branches make a soft natural yellow. Spinach makes a low-grade green dye.

Chop up the material in as small pieces as possible. Cover with water and boil over low heat for an hour.

All of these processes that require heat are best done in winter when the house can be warmed at the same time. All of the above colors are excellent for camouflage clothing.

Lye

All survivors will have a great need for lye. It is one of the key ingredients in many homemade products.

Lye is best made over a period of time. Problems that arise when hurrying the process won't occur if you take your time and plan ahead.

Start by burning a large rack of hardwood (it must be hardwood) down to ashes. If you burn nothing but hardwood in your stove, you can save that material for use in making lye.

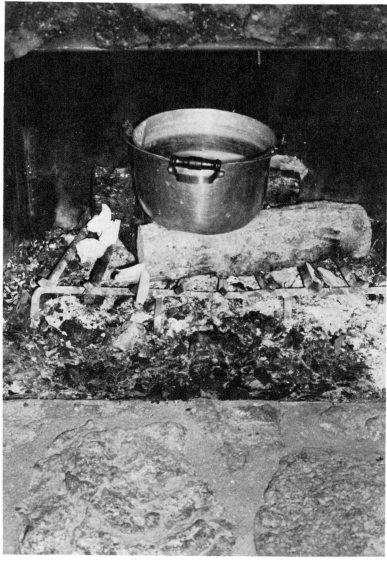

An oversize stainless steel kettle filled with boiling deer tallow and lye to produce soap. After boiling slowly for several hours, a spoonful of the mixture is dropped into cold water for testing. If it hardens properly, it is time to pour the mixture into old cupcake tins or paper tubes, or onto cookie sheets where it can harden and then be cut into pieces. Once the reader has obtained tallow and lye, soap is fairly easy to make, even with improvised equipment.

Use a large wooden barrel or if that is not possible, a plastic garbage can. Thirty gallons is about the minimum size that you should fool with. Drill about twenty-five ½-inch holes along the bottom edge of the barrel. Place the barrel on a rack with a pan or piece of plastic below to funnel the leach out to a 5-gallon pail. Place a layer of coarse dried grass along the bottom of the barrel for a filter.

Now pack the barrel solid with hardwood ashes. Don't use any ashes that have been rained on or otherwise wetted. The full basket or barrel will be quite heavy, and generally is best packed in place over the leaching rack.

I start by pouring three to five gallons of water on the ashes. Cover the barrel and allow the liquid to drain through for three days. Add more water at regular intervals till the liquid coming out the bottom no longer tastes bitter. The best leaching setup occurs in climates where the water collected in the bottom bucket evaporates about as fast as the water is added in the top. Over a period of weeks a total of about 15 gallons of water should be run through the 30 gallons of ash.

Gently boil the leached water down if evaporation isn't sufficient. When the process is completed the liquid should float a carrot or heavy potato right on top with no problem. Store the liquid in plastic bleach bottles for later use. Thirty gallons of ash makes about one gallon of lye.

Making Soap

Manufacture most of your soap in small batches. Use fats like beef or deer tallow for heavy laundry or floor washing soap, and lighter fats such as goat or even raccoon or possum for hand soap. Goose grease makes some of the best face soap going.

Take a gallon of lye produced using the previous instructions and bring it to a gentle boil. Add in fat till you have a thick, almost oatmeal-like mixture. Use an iron or stainless steel pot, never aluminum.

Boil this "soup" gently for two and a half hours and cool a sample to see if it will set up. If not, boil some more.

When the boiling soap is ready to set up, add about a tablespoon of salt per gallon and a chunk of rosin about the size of a quail's head. Don't add salt if you used salty pork fat as the fat ingredient.

LYE LEACHING SETUP

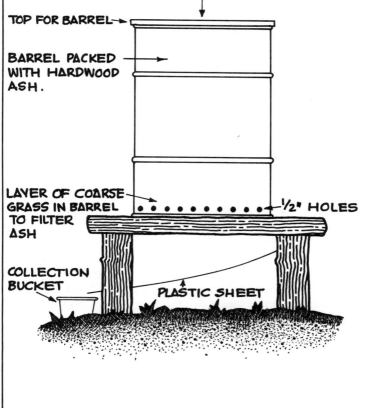

PLASTIC OR WOOD BARREL · MINIMUM 30 GAL.

TOP FOR BARREL →

BARREL PACKED WITH HARDWOOD ASH.

LAYER OF COARSE GRASS IN BARREL TO FILTER ASH

½" HOLES

COLLECTION BUCKET

PLASTIC SHEET

I make molds out of heavy paper and pour my liquid soap into these. Sometimes it is handy to mold a cord into the soap.

Experiment producing soap with various materials. It is not that difficult to make good personal and laundry soap. It's also possible to turn out some of grandma's old-fashioned "XXX" lye soap that will take your skin off with the dirt.

Deodorant and Perfume

Save and dry beaver castors for this purpose. A very small piece mixed in with your homemade soap is really quite nice. A chunk ground up and spread in a cloth is a great deodorizer in a house full of cooking cabbage, too. Beaver castor also makes good trapping lure. Foxes and coyotes come right to it.

Canvas Tent Waterproofing

Use deer tallow, beeswax, and white gasoline if you can get it. Mix a gallon of gas and 1 pound each of tallow and beeswax. Dissolve and apply to the tent with an old rag.

If no gasoline is available, mix lard and beeswax together over a gentle heat. Set the tent up in the warm sun and quickly apply the mixture as evenly as possible, while it is still liquid.

Soft Water

Collect rainwater using a large plastic tarp and a plastic waste-basket. Store it away quickly after the rain or the water will collect dirt as well. Rainwater is soft, or relatively free of dissolved minerals.

Leather Laces and Straps

Enlist a single-edged razor blade sharpened on a stone and strop to cut these. First make a single straight cut up the back line of the hide, separating it in two. This produces a straight line from which to begin slicing. Don't forget to plan out the cuts so the needed pieces aren't forgotten. As you work around the flanks, the leather gets thinner. Make wide thick straps from the top leather, shoelaces from the sides, and save the remainder for glove leather, for example.

Hold the razor between your thumb and forefinger and gauge the width of the cuts with the forefinger. For wider straps, use the social finger as a gauge.

Many times it works better if two people hold the skin taut, especially if laces are being made. Some light skins can be cut with a well-sharpened tin snips or poultry shears.

Vinegar

This is a product that will be needed in large quantities by survivalists.

It is possible to make fairly good vinegar from apple cider. Fresh apple juice will turn to vinegar if it is stored in glass bottles that are left sitting for a few days. At least once a day the cork must be opened to relieve the pressure and to let some air in. Mildly alcoholic hard cider will result if the juice is not allowed to breathe. The bottle may even blow up.

Serviceable vinegar can be made by pouring off half a jug of good vinegar into a second bottle. Add enough soft water to fill it again and 1 heaping cup of brown sugar. In about a week, depending on the temperature, the mixture will remake itself.

I don't know if this trick will work past three or four dilutions. Perhaps it will. We may soon have a good chance to find out.

Feather and Down Clothing

At present we save all the down and feathers from the ducks we raise and shoot to use as filling in down vests and pillows, and to replace worn-out filling in our sleeping bags. The only feathers we don't save are the very large wing feathers.

Pluck the ducks wet, the same as usual. As best as possible, sort the large feathers out and throw them away. Don't make a big deal about this procedure however, since it is certainly more important at the time to get the ducks cleaned.

The feathers should be allowed to accumulate on a clean cement or wood floor. After the plucking is finished, leave the feathers for a day or two. If they are very wet, rake them a bit to speed drying.

Collect the feathers in large paper sacks and staple shut. They will keep up to two years this way.

Cat Skin Gloves

An old tomcat has some of the toughest, most durable skin you will ever come across. One large cat usually has enough fur to make two mittens. If the weather is really cold, sew an exterior layer of buckskin to the cat skin liner for added protection.

Cat skin is a valuable resource. Don't overlook it.

Lamp Oil

Some fish are so full of oil that they can be put in a tin can, lit with a match, and used for light. Needlefish or Pacific smelt and some herring will work. Undoubtedly there are many other species that are similarly oily and will burn for light. You might do some checking around in your area.

Any fat that will stay liquid at low temperatures will work in lamps. Some of these are fat from seal, porpoise, coon, bear, possum, and groundhog. The simplest procedure is to take a piece of cotton cloth twisted into a wick and put it in a small bowl of oil. Light the wick and, behold, a small amount of light. In winter the lamp will heat the room slightly as well.

Candles

Lard and beeswax can be molded in paper tubes to make half-assed candles. It is a shameful waste of beeswax, but without paraffin, it's the only way I know of to make candles.

Use cotton cloth cut very thin and tightly twisted for a wick. Hang the wick in the center of the paper-tube mold. Melt the lard and the beeswax together in a 60:40 ratio and pour in the mold. Mutton or deer tallow works even better if you have either of these to add to the beeswax.

Neatsfoot Oil

Neatsfoot oil is made by slow-boiling hooves and hide trimmings in water for five to seven days. If whole hides are used, be sure to wash off the salt and cut into small pieces before boiling. Sometimes this is a very good use for old torn skins that otherwise have no value.

The hair does not have to be removed from the skin. After boiling a while, it will float to the surface. Then it can be skimmed for use in mortar, or for making cushions, or just left in the pot to boil away.

After all the pieces have disintegrated, boil another day before allowing the mixture to cool. As it cools, oil will come to the top. This is the neatsfoot oil that has so many uses.

Skim the oil off and store in bottles for later use. Unfortunately, a 20-gallon kettle of hides and hooves will yield at most 1 gallon of oil. Most of the remainders will be animal glue. Hopefully you will think of some good use for all the glue.

Indian Sleeping Bag

Occasionally I have young tinhorns ask me how the Indians got along without down-filled sleeping bags. Actually, the Indians had their own style of bedrolls, which were warmer than a three-pound down bag and only slightly heavier.

They saved all of their winter-caught rabbits and tanned perhaps one hundred fifty or more skins at one time. Generally they brain tanned, or used bark tanning. The tanned rabbit skins were trimmed square, doing away with most of the thin belly fur, legs, heads, and other irregular pieces. Not all the patches of skin were of equal size. Yet by sorting and matching, the Indians were able to sew together a blanket of solid skins roughly 6 feet square. All of the skins were sewn together very carefully with thousands of tiny stitches. The end product was very strong.

Next a layer of doe or fawn skin, heavy cloth, a facing layer of rabbit skins, groundhog leather, or whatever light leather was available was sewn against the fur-side of the bedroll. The purpose was to protect the rabbit fur from dirt and wet, and to provide a water-resistant outer layer. The exterior leather was lightly oiled.

The finished rabbit bedroll weighs in at about eight pounds. It will last two years under constant use, if timely repairs are made. Not using the roll is about as destructive as using it. They seem to deteriorate sitting around.

I believe a blanket of this type made from domestic winter-killed New Zealand white rabbits, backed with goat or light deerskin would last five years, and enable one to sleep comfortably on the ground in zero weather.

"Cat" Gut

In spite of what the name implies, the intestines of any animal can be used for gut lacing. Deer intestines are very good for this purpose.

Take the intestines out of the animal, as carefully as possible. No muscle tissue should be left with the guts. Split down one side and clean in water. Hang the cleaned gut over a line and let dry. Once dehydrated, the gut will keep for ten years. When you want to use it, throw the gut in a pan of water for a day or two and allow it to soften.

This material is ideal to repair a table leg, for instance. While the gut is wet, wind it around the break. It will dry so hard nothing will move it.

Deer Hair

Use the leftover hair from your tannery operation in mortar. It makes the stuff two or three times stronger.

Horns

Sliced in thin pieces and drilled, horn makes ideal buttons. It is also a reasonably good replacement for bakelight pot and pan handles.

Porkypine Quills

Dried, the large quills make fair leather awls. They can also be used to sew with in an emergency.

16. Bees and Honey

It is quite possible that bees could become our primary source for sweetening after a collapse and all the traditional sources of commercial sugar have dried up. But honey is not the only product bees produce—they also provide us with a much needed service. Without bees to pollinate our fruit and vegetable plants, there wouldn't be much of a crop. Beeswax rendered down from the comb is another valuable product. There are hundreds of uses for it—everything from lubricating thread prior to sewing leather, to rustproofing, to sealing jars of jam, to patching a water bucket.

My first experience with bees was as a young boy in the capacity of a "hunter," for I spent countless hours hunting for wild bee trees that I could raid for the honey and wax.

At one time bee hunting was a popular outdoor pastime in this country. During the late fall it was common to see the old woodsmen out with their bait, scent, and catch boxes trying to "get a line on a bee." Indian summer, when it was still warm enough for the bees to fly, was and still is the best time for bee hunting. The little critters are hungry then, and readily come to a bait.

Little did I know that the skills I learned back then were part of a dying art. To the best of my knowledge, there hasn't been an article written on bee hunting for the last thirty years. I doubt if there are more than a handful of skilled bee hunters left in the entire U.S. and Canada.

Bee hunting as a recreational outdoor activity passed into history as a result of two unrelated effects of civilization. Most of our native bees were domesticated, and large tracts of forest were cleared.

During the 1920s and 1930s it was usual for beekeepers to expand their colonies by collecting wild bees. They would locate wild swarms of black bees and transfer them into portable beehives. All of the hives were transported to a central area where they were watched and cared for much like domestic livestock.

Once the new bee colony was safely under control by the keeper, he would remove the wild black queen and replace her with a yellow-banded Italian variety. The life span of a bee is four months at the most. During the active honey season, the workers often last only thirty days or less. By replacing the queen who in turn laid all of the eggs for the colony, the apiarist effectively wiped out the original wild swarm. The original black bees disappeared, victims of normal attrition.

Two phenomena developed as a result. A large percentage of the wild colonies were captured, and in turn were converted to a more docile, domestic species of yellow bee.

The other consequence of civilization—clearing of many forests, especially the eastern hardwoods—reduced the number of trees available for bees. Before very long, the situation came to a head. Old-timers like myself remember that eventually, the only bees that came to a bait anymore were actually domestic kinds that were already living in somebody's hive.

The Bee Colony

There are three kinds of bees in a colony. Most numerous and often encountered are the workers. These are the smallest. A few drones are present in every colony. They are the intermediate-sized bee, larger than workers but much smaller than the queen. Large numbers of drones in a hive indicate that something is amiss, usually that the queen has become infertile.

The only function of the drones is to provide a mate for the recently hatched queen. The ever-tidy workers keep a few around. In fall when the food supply dwindles, they will kill off almost all the nonworking drones.

The queen is the economic center and ruler of the hive. She busies herself laying eggs, carefully regulating the supply of new workers to match the available food supply. She is the largest bee in the group, often the hardest to spot. She is only one of many and is covered and protected by all the bees around her.

Bees collect nectar and manufacture honey as a means of providing food for the colony over winter. Being very industrious, they often process five to ten times as much honey as will be needed. During the winter they propagate themselves at a greatly reduced rate, conserving their food supplies. When spring comes, the queen will lay thousands of extra eggs to enlarge the population of the colony. This provides workers for the coming harvest.

If there are abundant flowers, the queen will continue to expand the population of the hive. The workers, noting the plentiful harvest, also react. They may begin a special sixteen-day feeding cycle to produce an additional queen. When the hive gets too crowded, some workers will follow the newly produced queen to different quarters, leaving an old queen and perhaps half the workers behind to keep the old colony going. Wherever the new queen stops the workers will land and hang on her, or do what we refer to as "swarming."

Bees by nature are very prolific. Portions of a healthy colony will swarm at least once and sometimes twice each year, if the conditions are right. Nothing is wasted. They will reproduce fast enough to use all of the available crop. If there are lots of flowers, they will definitely swarm twice.

Back to the Wild

Often domestic swarms of bees will get away from their keeper and take off into the wild. There they find a hollow tree in which to take up permanent residence. With the coming of today's second-growth timber there are again sufficient places where such bees can hive. Italian bees have adapted well to our climate, providing the strong stock needed to reestablish colonies in the wild. The only force acting against the spread of wild bees back to their natural habitat is the widespread use of insecticides in some areas.

When to Harvest

Often I have located colonies in the spring, when the bees are sluggish and weak from their winter dormancy. Never, under any circumstances have I cut the tree or otherwise disturbed them at that time. During spring, even bees in town are best left living in the side of a building, or in the backyard apple tree where you found them.

Waiting till late fall to harvest the honey can also be disastrous for the bees, unless special precautions are taken. Either early in the season or at the close of it in fall, if you take their food and destroy their home, there is nothing for the bees to do but die. Killing colonies of bees is not in the reader's best interest.

My policy is to leave the bees alone in spring. After they have collected honey all summer, I may cut the tree in fall if a hive box is available to transfer the bees into.

Judging from my experience hunting bees, I feel that there are more wild bees today than there have been for at least forty years. This is good news for the survivalist who will probably have to rely on bees for the principal source of his domestic sweets.

"Lining" Wild Bees

Wild bee trees are found using one of several methods that are all known as "lining." All require a great deal of skill and patience, but are so interesting that I often spend way too much time at it. Like a good piece of jazz, there is often more than one good way to handle it. Sometimes one lining method works better and other times another method may work. You might have a lot of fun going out and giving it a whirl.

Bee trees can be hunted from the first few days in spring, till the last warm days of Indian summer. Philosophically, it doesn't matter when they are hunted as long as the honey is not taken at the wrong time. Since bees will come in to bait more easily when they are hungry, most hunters go out in early spring or late fall.

Colonies of bees generally locate in hollow, rotten parts of live standing trees. They may also be found in old buildings, abandoned commercial hives, in downed logs, or even in a hole in the rocks or ground.

Bees do not fly in a "beeline." Often they will fly in protected draws or along fence lines to escape head winds. The home tree may be half a mile away, but they may fly one mile to get there. The following are some methods I use to establish a line by using bait.

In early spring or late fall, bees can be lured over long distances by burning honeycomb. This can be done on a previously heated flat rock, or over a small camp stove. Using the camp stove, heat up a coffee can red-hot and throw in a piece of honey-filled comb that has been soaked in water. Turn off the fire and allow the wax and honey to turn to steam and smoke. Heated rocks are removed from the campfire and set on a stump or other convenient place. Throw the water-soaked comb on the rock the same as with the hot coffee can.

Bees can also be attracted to an area using a few drops of pure clove oil worked into a clean rag. Put the rag up in a tree or on a pole at first to get wider exposure.

Soon bees will be heard zooming around looking for the food. Keep them coming by putting some fresh green shrub branches over the now-cooling rock and sprinkling liberally with bait. I make my bait out of one part honey, one part sugar, and two parts clean water. Don't use city water with chlorine in it.

Another method of starting bees on bait is by using either a drinking glass or a catch box.

Use the glass to catch a bee on a flower or at a watering place. Put a piece of cardboard under the glass and take the bee back to the bait. This can be the mixture on brush, or a piece of fresh comb. Put the upside-down glass over the bait and remove the cardboard. By shading the glass it is possible to get the bee down on the bait, as it tries to stay in the light. Soon it will start feeding on the free grits, and the glass can be removed.

Keep catching bees and putting them on the bait till a strong flight between the hive and bait is established.

Catch boxes are small wooden containers about twice the size of large wooden matchboxes. They have two separate boxes. The bottom one holds some bait and has a sliding top. The top box has a sliding bottom door with a screen top so you can see what is happening inside. These devices are hard to build. That's one reason few people use them; I have never seen them for sale.

Using the baited catch box, the bee hunter collects as many bees as practical and takes them back to the main bait. The catch-and-carry process should be repeated enough times to establish a flight of bees from the bait to the hive.

At times this may occur very rapidly. Other times it may be three or four hours till a strong line of bees can be established: Bee hunting is good enough in most parts of the country that there are often three to five different lines, indicating that at least that many different colonies are working the bait.

I draw a simple diagram showing the direction and intensity of the flights if there are three or more. This saves starting the catch-and-bait procedure up again later, should seeking out one hive take more than a day or two.

Baiting should be done in a clearing or open area where the view of the departing bees is as unrestricted as possible. Depending on the season and the condition of the flowers, bees will travel as far as two miles for food.

After a line is established, I pick the strongest course and move off as far as I can in the direction of the bees' travel to a place where I am still able to see or hear their line. Sometimes it is possible to run after the bees for a considerable distance before they drop from sight.

The next part of the finding procedure requires a good deal of common sense.

Trap as many bees as possible in the catch box and move the bait and box with bees along the direction of the line. If no bait box is being used, move the bait-covered branches, or the piece of comb if that is what was used. Set up again, as far as you think practical, along the observed, route of flight. Reestablish the flights by either burning bait, using scent, or catching bees. Hopefully this should not take a great deal of time.

Catch boxes are more practical to make a move with. Just be careful the bees are trapped away from the main bait, or they will take an hour to clean themselves before starting to work again.

Flights out of the second station should be stronger in the initial direction you are working, and much thinner in other directions. This is assuming there are more than one flight, and the move you made was in the correct direction of the hive.

Keep working the lines of flight, following them as much as possible. Sometimes it helps to sprinkle a tiny bit of flour on a few bees. If the light is right they can be seen at greater distances.

Bee activity will drop off to nothing if a move takes you past the hive. If that happens, go back to the last bait station and search the route of flight more diligently. Make a shorter move.

Bee activity will pick up dramatically near the hive. Within one hundred yards of the tree, there should be a constant stream that is easy to follow.

Transferring Bees

Transferring wild bees to a hive is tricky, but not nearly as difficult as the novice might first suspect.

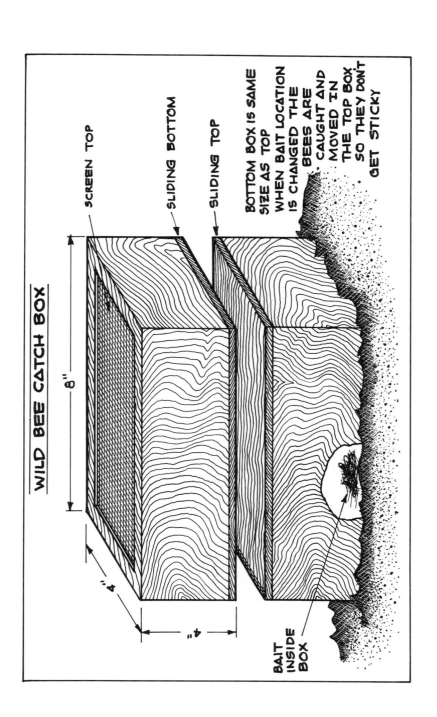

WILD BEE CATCH BOX

SCREEN TOP

SLIDING BOTTOM

SLIDING TOP

BOTTOM BOX IS SAME
SIZE AS TOP
WHEN BAIT LOCATION
IS CHANGED THE
BEES ARE
CAUGHT AND
MOVED IN
THE TOP BOX
SO THEY DON'T
GET STICKY

BAIT
INSIDE
BOX

8"

8"

4"

The Achilles' heel of the average bee is its propensity to fill up on honey when seriously disturbed. Having done so, the bees are relatively harmless. They either can't or won't sting! Surprise, surprise. Now you know how beekeepers can safely handle the massive swarms of bees you often see them with in pictures.

Some bee hunters and keepers go about their work without any protective covering. I use an old army surplus mesquito headnet, a pair of thin leather gloves, a nylon shell jacket, and a pair of medium-weight cotton pants.

The only other piece of equipment that is at all specialized for transferring bees is a smoker. My suggestion is to buy one from Sears. They are just too damn much trouble to make at home.

Smokers are used to frighten the bees, causing them to load up with honey. Fuel is an old piece of denim, burlap sack, or even a few dry leaves. Practice a bit with the thing ahead of time to be sure you know how to make it smoke.

During midsummer, wild colonies can often be raided without transferring the bees to a hive or killing them. The trick is to take only a small portion of the honeycomb, damaging the brood comb and hive as little as possible. The bees will find a new place to live if they and the queens remain basically intact. By cold weather the industrious little guys are often reestablished in good shape.

Sometimes it is possible to collect honey from a wild colony without cutting down the tree. I have done this by taking out a section of the log and replacing it when I was done. The bees didn't like it, but soon life was back to normal.

Sometimes it may be necessary to raid a colony in such a way that its death is certain. Usually this happens when one tries to move an established group of bees out of a wall or building in town. The old-fashioned method is to use a burning torch. Simply rile the bees and burn their wings off as they come out of the building. In the past I have also used a CO_2 fire extinguisher to freeze them out.

Here's the very best way I know of for moving a wild nest of bees from a tree into a domestic hive. Start by using a saw to cut the tree off right above the wild hive. During the cutting, worker bees will become frightened, and gorge on honey. They cluster around their queen, and become relatively passive. After the top of the wild hive is exposed you must reach in and transfer the mass of bees to your commercial hive. Seal the commercial hive before transporting it to your final destination.

All of the honeycomb within the now-deserted tree hive should be removed immediately. Otherwise, robber bees will carry it off.

Processing Honeycomb

Comb from wild bees is mixed. Some of it is brood comb and some contains honey. The only practical method of separating the two is by hand, laying aside the real dirty, woody stuff for bait or feed. If possible, set aside some of the very clean honeycomb to be eaten whole. Basically, however, almost all of it goes into a large pot to be rendered.

Honey should be rendered over a very low, even heat. Don't hurry or it will burn. After everything has melted, while the mixture is still warm, skim off the floating "bee's knees." The wax is valuable. Leave as much as possible when skimming the bee's knees flotsam.

Allow the mixture to chill, or at least cool. Carefully slice the wax layer free of the pot and remove. I recast my beeswax into convenient cakes in old cupcake tins.

The honey below the layer of wax should be stored in smaller jars. It keeps nicely in quart jars with screw-on lids.

Commercial Beehives

Commercial beehives look simple to the casual observer. Yet there is an amazing amount of practical engineering in each one. Every feature is incorporated for a precise reason. Possibly you can learn to build beehives at home, but initially I don't recommend it. Would-be beekeepers need to look at the correct equipment first, before striking out on their own. Now, while it is still possible, buy premade hives from Sears. Later you may want to build from scratch, after you know what to build.

Starting at the bottom, the hive must first have a solid raised base. The base is closed in back and has a movable bottom bar in the front. Bottom bars are blocks of wood that restrict the size of the hive opening.

A 20-by-16-by-9½-inch brood chamber sits directly on the base. Inside are from six to ten frames. Brood chamber and frames

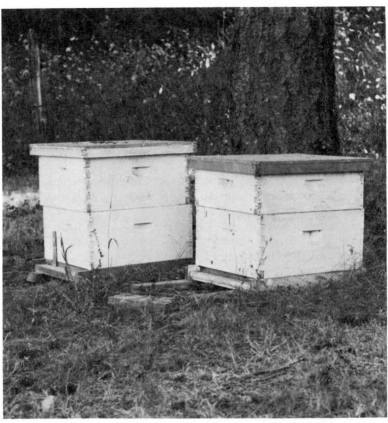

Two domestic beehives located on the author's retreat. If possible, readers should learn how to raise bees. A modest colony can produce fifty pounds of honey per year, which is enough for a large family for an entire year, with some left over for barter stock. These hives are secured for the winter. The lower section in each hive contains the main colony of bees; the top sections are supers, full of honey for the bees' winter needs. The beekeeper will later add as many as four or five supers to be filled by the workers as the summer progresses.

must be purchased as a unit to ensure that they fit together correctly.

Generally if it is available, I put commercial comb foundation in my frames. The bees get a better start when they don't have to make the comb from scratch. Also the comb foundation directs their efforts into more orderly, neat comb construction.

Always use double lids with telescoping covers to cap the hive. No water, snow, sand or anything else should get through from the top. Commercial covers are always lined with metal or fiberglass.

After the bees get established, they will form the comb and fill it with honey and brood. This should happen fairly soon after the bees have been moved into the hive.

Be very careful not to let your bees get crowded. As soon as it looks like they may fill the lower chamber, start adding what are known as "supers."

There are three sizes of supers. Two sizes are smaller than the brood chamber and one is the same size. Each super comes with a set of ten frames that should be filled with comb foundation. These supers are what the bees fill with honey as they expand the stores of the colony. To avoid inventory problems I use the one size of super that is also the same size as the brood chamber.

Keep supers free of brood comb by laying a wire excluder on top of the brood chamber. Only the workers with honey can get through the wire into the top supers. During the winter the bee-keeper may want to take the excluder out so all the bees can get something to eat. This is assuming the supplies in the main chamber run out.

I have had second- and third-year colonies produce four big supers full of honey. That is more sweetening than we need for the entire year, including cooking, baking, and canning.

The importance of honey to the survivalist is obvious. Yet it seems to me that few people will be prepared to find and cultivate the bees necessary to provide what they need. I find the entire process of lining and propagating bees to be extremely interesting. Perhaps you will share this interest. It will make self-sufficiency a bunch easier to achieve.

17. Practical Domestic Animals

The Nez Perce amply demonstrated that in a subsistence life-style, the standard of living can be greatly improved through the raising of domestic animals. This is not to say that the Nez Perce was the only tribe who kept domestic or semidomestic animals around. But they were the only tribe to develop selective breeding techniques that allowed them to improve their stock. All other Indians allowed their stock to breed at random, even if it degenerated to the point of having less utilitarian value.

Domestic stock for the survivalist or retreater is not the same thing as domestic stock under our present economy. Actually the term *semidomestic* would be more specific. These are animals that more or less take care of themselves. They can provide you with food and clothing products, but find most of the food they need without much human help.

Dogs and guinea fowl have already been mentioned as two possibilities. The additional five I am going to cover do not comprise an exhaustive list. They are merely examples of animals I or my family have raised in a survival situation, and found to be practical.

Rabbits

My long-departed parents would roll over in their graves if I didn't start this chapter with a section on domestic rabbits. My dad often talked about raising rabbits on his porch in Germany during World War I. After the truce and the ensuing financial collapse, they traded rabbits for potatoes and raised cabbage. That was all they had to eat.

My mother was a young girl in Russia when the Summer Revolution of 1905 broke out. Their small farm implement business was burned and they personally were driven out of town. Mother used to tell about raising rabbits in small pens, feeding them grass, and making do on the meat they provided.

Rabbits are fairly prolific, relatively easy to keep, and will exist on nothing more than fresh grass, hay, and salt. Usually they are kept in wire or slat pens measuring about 3 feet by 2 feet by 2 feet. The does require a wooden nest box that they can enter easily. In very severe winters, all of the rabbits will need a nest box plus some sort of overhead shelter. The porch of a house is a fine place for rabbits if the roof is tight and the hutches can be backed against a solid wall.

Rabbits breed at ten months of age, bearing eight to ten young after a thirty-day gestation. Older does will bear ten to fourteen young. They generally remain in good breeding shape for about four years.

One buck will breed five does if the breedings are spaced apart rather than bunched together. Commercial breeders like to have all the young come at one time. Even if there are as few as five does, the owner should keep an extra buck in case something happens to the regular buck.

At times, rabbits are really tough to get to breed. If the winters are very cold, or the food old and stale, it is virtually impossible. In general, the most even an experienced rabbit raiser can expect is about three litters a year.

Breed does should be kept in peace and seclusion. Don't rile them up, especially right after they have their young.

Rabbits are weaned at six weeks and generally slaughtered any time after nine weeks. Keeping them past sixteen weeks is counterproductive unless there is a need for replacement breeding stock. Does are rebred at nine weeks, if possible.

The best domestic rabbits, in my estimation, are the big white kind. Their skins are large and heavy, and easy to make into gloves and blankets.

I hang my rabbit pens on a wall and let the droppings fall through the wire bottom. Periodically we collect the droppings for use as fertilizer in the garden.

Don't ever feed rabbits wet grass. They will get diarrhea from it and die. Dried clover or alfalfa is best in winter, although properly dried lawn clippings are almost as good.

For a time when we lived in the South, we let our domestic rabbits run wild in a large two-acre yard. The only thing keeping them in was a low, two-foot chicken wire fence. It was a nice situation. The rabbits took care of themselves, and even mowed our grass a bit.

They also proliferated tremendously. Our biggest problem turned out to be trapping them. They wouldn't go in box traps, and were tough to catch in snares. Later in winter it was much easier to catch them, since they got hungry and came to bait. Occasionally we shot some, but this was a poor practice. There was too much chance of killing a doe with a litter.

Initially the only predators were stray dogs, cats, and an occasional owl. All became familiar with the crack of my .25-.20. As an added bonus, some coons and foxes started coming in. My wife caught the foxes in steel traps.

Twenty breeding does will produce enough meat and fur to keep a family of four going. Rabbits are good critters for city dwellers to raise, unless everyone else decides to raise them as well and all the grass disappears. Their diseases are few, they don't smell, and they are easy to handle.

Carp

I really don't care a great deal for eating carp, but they do merit a place in this chapter. Carp reproduce rapidly, grow to a fairly good size in a short period of time, and eat vegetative matter that nothing else will. They will thrive in any halfway clean pond that doesn't freeze solid in winter.

If you have a small fished-out pond nearby, you might give some thought to stocking it with carp. They can live under conditions unsuitable to other species. In the last thirty years, I have stocked two formerly barren farm ponds with carp. In both cases the fish grew rapidly and reproduced well. I don't know what they ate. It wasn't anything I gave them. But be aware that carp can quickly take over a pond, pushing out more desirable fish.

I originally put the carp in the ponds to give the kids some big fish to catch that wouldn't particularly tax their fishing ability. In five years we had dozens of six-pound fish. Some eventually got bigger, but they were the exception. The kids caught hundreds of these carp without ever denting the population.

Pond depths of about six feet seem about right for carp. Perhaps they could be raised in shallower ponds. Remember that the cleaner and fresher the water, the better the fish will taste.

If the carp are harvested in fish traps, they can be returned unharmed to grow some more. Cut a small piece out of the fin when you do. By tagging them this way, it is possible to keep track of their growth rate.

Goats

In the Bible, the goat is used as a symbol of the devil. And indeed they behave like the very devil. Wherever goats are left to fend for themselves, they girdle trees, kill the native foliage, and generally raise hell.

In my opinion, goats have rather tasteless meat, the exception being the old billies that can get awfully rank as they grow older. My suggestion is to plan way ahead and keep virtually all the male goats castrated.

One of the principal reasons for keeping goats is that they will eat weeds and brush and take care of themselves. In the bargain, they become quite wild. Sometimes the only way to catch up with one is to shoot it. Since a billy shouldn't be eaten before it has lived at least six months without its testicles, this can be a problem.

There are several ways to handle this situation. You can provide a barn or shed where they go for shelter and catch them in there, run down the very young kids shortly after birth, or snare the goats and catch them that way.

A nanny goat will breed at about ten months and usually have a single offspring. After that they usually have twins or triplets. Breeding stock is generally good through about six years.

Nothing much will bother a herd of goats. Even coyotes seem afraid of them.

I try to keep track of my stock even if it is loose and running around a thick bayou or wooded area. That way I can keep up with some sort of a selective breeding program. Since goats live on grass, weeds, and bushes, it usually isn't difficult to keep them around, and simply butcher one when the meat supply is low. Often they will browse through even a rough winter without any additional feed from the owner.

Goats, as a practical matter, are about the biggest domestic animals that a city survivor would ever want to keep. This can work well if you've got enough grass and weeds around to feed them. They also may need to be tied to a leash, or you'll never see them again.

Some folks milk their goats. I never needed the milk that badly, so I always let the young goats have it. After the kids are weaned, the nanny must be milked twice a day, or she will go dry. This ties one down to a degree that I have never liked.

Goat skins make incredibly tough glove leather, and very nice vests. Some people might raise them just for their skins.

Ducks

A lot of classic survivalists suggest raising chickens. It is my contention that these folks have never tried raising chickens or they wouldn't make such an asinine proposal. Chickens must be the dumbest birds in the world. They can barely take care of themselves, often reproduce poorly, are subject to many diseases, and fall victim to a wide range of predators.

Ducks, on the other hand, are none of the above.

White Pekin ducks are not very good "setters," or egg layers. But Rouens and Muskovy ducks are good setters and good mothers. They all lay as many eggs as chickens but duck eggs are much larger and better tasting.

Ducks will set twice if allowed to hatch the first clutch early. If you want a second hatch, take the day-old ducklings away and raise them yourself.

A typical hatch contains twelve to fifteen young, and takes about thirty-five days. Breeding ducks should be kept through the third year.

Ducks never get sick that I know of, and have few predators. I let mine run loose in the yard. They are very good about staying where they belong and keeping out of trouble. Sometimes foxes or coyotes make a try for them. Up till now the dogs have always kept them away.

The biggest single advantage of ducks over chickens is their ability to do a better job of scrounging food. They eat a much wider range of things than almost any other bird, and are much neater

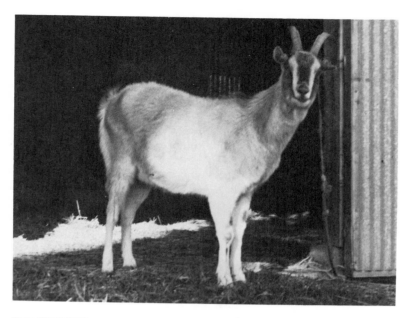

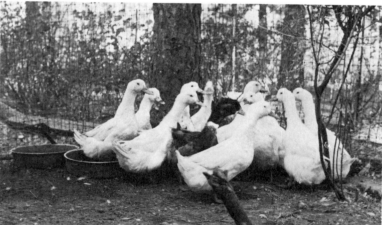

Top: Goats are ideal practical animals for the survivalist to keep at home or retreat. They require little care, will eat foliage no other animal will touch, and seldom get sick. Be warned that goats can be mean!

Bottom: Domestic ducks are another first choice for the survivalist. They have the same good traits that goats do, plus ducks can provide eggs, feathers and down, and rendered fat. The author strongly favors domestic ducks over chickens.

doing it. Our ducks keep a significant amount of the lawn eaten down so that it requires little mowing.

In winter, ducks must be fed. They survive cold much better than any other bird I know of, but still require a small amount of supplementary grain.

Other than meat, ducks produce a fine grade of cooking and waterproofing oil, and feather and down that make nice pillows, comforters, and vests.

Sometimes in spring ducks won't start laying. I solve this by hanging a lantern out in their pen to attract bugs. When the ducks are hyped by extra protein, the eggs start to roll.

By far and away the biggest problem with ducks is the smell. When crowded, it is awesome. I get around this by limiting the number I keep and by restricting the amount of water they have.

With sufficient space, ducks are an absolute delight. They are even semi-intelligent.

Pigeons

I have eaten so many pigeons that I can't stand them anymore. But they are good animals for the survivalist, so deserve a mention in that regard.

The principal advantage of a pigeon over many other animals is that they require absolutely no work or care. They will fly out and find all of their own food. If you will have to make it in the city, pigeons are an especially good bet. Seventy-five or so can provide about 25 percent of a family's meat needs, at no cost to the owner.

After the collapse it is my feeling that pigeons will proliferate in the big cities. They will live in the then-unoccupied highrise buildings, sallying forth to feed on the weed seeds that will be abundant.

The reader could go into the pigeon business by finding a dimly lit loft or attic that the pigeons can get into. It may be necessary to break a window or board up all but one window to make the place suitable.

Roost boards should be nailed up high near the ceiling for the pigeons to build their nests on. They must be at least six inches wide.

To get the pigeons started, live-trap as many as possible and coop them up in your room. You will have to give them food and water, and you may as well eat the old birds. They will never come back after you once turn them loose.

After three weeks, allow the pigeons to start flying, but keep on feeding them for another two weeks at least.

Pigeons mate and nest two or three times a year. Eat the grown males as soon as possible, plus any of the old females that show little inclination to raise a brood.

The loft area will become a filthy, smelly hole. There isn't much that can be done about that.

Harvest the pigeons at night by spotting with a light and grabbing them. Try to be selective, and disrupt them as little as you can.

There are many other animals that could be listed. Some, like sheep, hamsters, muskrats, and hogs might be a good bet for you, depending on your own situation. No matter who you are or where you are, give some thought to animals you can raise to supplement your diet, and then get started learning how to raise them.

18. A Survival Generator

A realistic, practical survival program virtually dictates the need for some electrical energy. As I have tried to point out over and over again, those who go to the woods expecting to eat berries and dig roots ain't going to make it. If they do survive, their lives will be so miserable it won't be worth it.

True survival, in the long run, requires a great deal of preparation and planning. The will to live, to make it, must be there, both to provide the impetus needed to prepare now, and to handle the tremendous amount of work one will have to accomplish to survive in style during a long-term disaster.

Having lived on the fringe of survival situations most of my years, I have concluded that, while life without electricity is certainly possible, it will be much more austere and grim than if some small amount of power is available. One of the first improvements we made on the farm was to install an electric delco system, but not to power a radio or vacuum sweeper. We put the system in so we could pump water for the livestock and for the house, and so we had a little light during the evening to use while canning beans, working hides, or otherwise doing the things necessary to stay alive.

The simple addition of just a small amount of electricity added immeasurably to our well-being, and to our ability to face what was often an imposing and hostile world.

Later in life we repeated the pattern several times. In Africa I put up a giant windmill with twelve-foot rotor, and our life in Wyoming started with the purchase of an Onan generator.

The need for emergency power generation has always been there, but until recently there were few options available to the survivalists. Larger diesel units, popular on remote farms, logging camps, and as emergency standby units in hospitals and office buildings, were impractical. They were far too costly to purchase for most people, but more important, the cost of operation was astronomical. Larger power plants burn gallons of fuel an hour and require constant maintenance.

Smaller, camper-type units in the 2,000 to 5,000 kilowatt range are not expensive to purchase, but are impractical to own. No matter if they are made by Honda, Yamaha, or in the U.S. by Pincor, all are lightly built units that run on regular gasoline. Their life and practicality is therefore extremely limited.

Choice of Fuel

The first, most important consideration when putting a generator package together is what the power source will be. As I mentioned earlier, there have been several occasions when I used alternate power sources. Wind and water are two examples. There is nothing wrong with using a windmill or turbine to produce electrical power, under the right conditions.

Just remember that electricity is tough to store. If the wind does not blow or the water run when you need power for the freezer or a few lights, your natural generator may not be worth a damn. Storage batteries are expensive to buy and maintain. I don't recommend them unless you are a good practical electrical engineer with a basement full of spare parts.

Alternate energy generators deteriorate rapidly when not in use. If conditions are good for this type of unit in your area, put one in on a co-generation basis with the power company as a partner. Then run it continually. By so doing, you will keep the unit maintained in good order against the day of dire need and it might even pay for itself with the energy it produces.

For the last twenty or so years I have been looking for a good little steam engine—one that is small enough to move around, is relatively inexpensive, has sufficient power, and is easy to.maintain. Back when I started my research, a hardheaded old farmer who had used steam tractors to plow with in the old days told me my criteria violated at least one law of thermodynamics and several economic laws. I have reluctantly concluded that he was correct. There ain't no such engine.

For the average survivalists like ourselves, this leaves a choice of one. It has to be a small diesel engine.

Diesels' advantages over gasoline are obvious. They burn from a third to a half less fuel, the engines last far longer than a gas version, are easier to maintain, use a variety of fuels, and the fuel is storable.

I have buried on my property a 1,000-gallon diesel and fuel oil tank that I keep filled to the top all the time. When we built our home/retreat, we decided to use oil as a back-up for our wood stoves. When it gets below zero, the burner kicks on, giving the house an extra shot of warmth.

My plan, in a survival situation, is to close off most of the house, heat it with wood, and save the fuel oil for the generator. Unlike gasoline that will deteriorate in a year or less, my 1,000 gallons of fuel oil will last for five years or more, if need be. It also burns nicely in my diesel generators, of course.

After that time, if the economy has not reverted to a more favorable situation, I can always look towards light vegetable oils for a diesel fuel source. At the rate of fuel consumption small diesel engines have, growing one's own vegetable fuel is entirely practical.

Locating a Small Diesel Engine

Until very recently, it has been difficult to locate a small diesel engine in the U.S. The ones available were made in Japan, Germany, or England. All were costly and bulky to handle. Few came in the small 7 to 10 horsepower range I needed.

Within the last year, the Jack Bryant firm in Turner, Oregon, has started importing small, inexpensive diesel engines made in mainland China. They range in size from 4 up to about 20 horsepower. Apparently the units are used to power small tractors in China. Jack Bryant sells them in the U.S. to pump water, run compressors, power golf carts and, of course, run generators.

Prices run from about seven hundred dollars for the smaller sizes up to seventeen hundred dollars for the 20 hp models. Power ratings are conservative. Most gasoline 4,000 kw generators, for instance, are powered with 10 hp gasoline engines. Bryant recommends a 7 horse-rated Chinese engine for the same size generator.

All of the various sizes and types of engines appear to be made in different Chinese factories. Since it is impossible to predict in which factory they were made, Byrant simply refers to them all as Chinese engines.

Each unit comes with a detailed instruction manual printed in Chinese, Russian, and, thankfully, English. Using the book to repair and service the engine is easy. It's all there in one-two-three-four style, simplified so that a common peasant in Mongolia can make repairs.

The engines themselves are extremely plain-looking, straight-forward, simple units. Exterior finish is adequate. Internally, the tolerances are as good or better than anything on the market. Although they haven't been in our country long enough to verify, the claim is that these engines will last about twenty thousand hours, or twenty to twenty-five years. Just to be sure, the manufacturer includes a teak box filled with spare valves, injector nozzles, rings, filters, gaskets, springs, bearings, and the tools necessary to install the parts. I would estimate there are at least two hundred dollars worth of extra goodies included in the purchase price of the basic unit.

Except for the larger models, the engines are crank-started. This is not a handicap except during the coldest winter when it is necessary to first warm the fuel, or add a small amount of gasoline to the fuel, or use ether to get things moving.

The large 20-horse engine is a two-cylinder model. All of the smaller models are single cylinder with large flywheel. Cooling is provided by a water evaporation tank on the top of the engine. This system could be used to heat water or to warm a room as a bonus to the power generated.

Breaking in the engine is not required. The factory assumes you may not do this correctly, so they take care of it for you. All the user has to do is take the engine out of the box, fill the crank case with 30-weight oil, the cooling system with water, the tank with fuel and start it up.

The Correct Number of Watts

This is an important consideration for the survivor. A unit that is too small could be dangerously disappointing. One that is too large will rob funds needed for other supplies, and will use too much precious fuel when the time comes to press it into service.

The important concept to remember is that you, the survivalist, must plan to get along after the crash. Getting along does not mean you will run your home like nothing has happened. It means you must determine what is absolutely essential and plan to provide at that level.

In my case, the most pressing need is going to be pumping water from our 225-foot well for ourselves, the animals, and the garden. Take a look at the chart—it shows pump sizes versus watts:

Motor hp	Watts to Start	Watts to Run
1/6	600	275
1/4	1,050	400
1/2	1,800	600
3/4	2,300	850
1	3,100	1,000
1 1/2	3,600	1,600

We have a one-horse pump. Note that it will take 3,100 watts to start a motor of that size, but only 1,000 watts to keep it running. A good rule of thumb is to always start the largest motor first and then let it run a minute before cutting in other electric appliances.

My second priority is my two freezers. They require about 1,200 watts to start and 400 watts each to run.

After that I may want to run a saw (800 watts), or a drill (1,000 watts), a radio (1,200 watts), some lights (300 watts) or a grinder (1,000 watts). Yet I don't have to run all of these at the same time I am pumping water or freezing food. It's simple to do one and then the other.

An electric stove, water heater, or room heater could use up to 10,000 watts or more. Obviously it is impractical to generate electricity with which to heat. No provision should be made in that regard.

Having considered all my power requirements, I have settled on a 4,000-watt generator driven by a 7 hp slow-speed Chinese diesel engine. This outfit does a very adequate job for me, costs less than sixteen hundred dollars, will last longer than I will and, best of all, burns about one liter of fuel an hour.

In actual tests I can pump all of the water we need and freeze all of the food we can use, on a hot August day, using a half-gallon of diesel fuel or less. During the winter, fuel consumption falls to half of that. We estimate we have enough diesel fuel stored underground to last a minimum of four years. At the end of that time, if our country hasn't learned its lesson and gone back to producing, I will plan on raising and making my own diesel-vegetable fuel.

Each reader will have to estimate his own minimal power needs. Many power consumption charts exist, or you can call Jack Bryant in Turner, Oregon. He is used to helping out survivalists, and can make realistic recommendations.

Of course, it isn't necessary to buy a 1,000-gallon oil tank. Three 55-gallon barrels of fuel will last almost a year, providing a cushion, while you start your new life as a survivor. Barrels of diesel fuel are easily and safely stored in a garage or shed. They won't spoil, and you can add to your stock as space and finances permit.

Building the Generator Unit

Assembling the components of a generator into an efficient unit is not especially difficult. Or, if there is no one around to weld up the simple little rack for you, Jack Bryant will do the job for a modest sum. My carrying rack is made out of secondhand 1-inch angle iron I was able to scrounge at the junk yard. Wheels came from a kid's tricycle.

Both the engine and the generator have convenient mounting brackets. Best here to mount the engine and the generator on uni-strut (available from electrical supply houses) so that the pulleys can be precisely aligned.

Chinese engines come in both 3,000 RPM high-speed models and low-speed 2,000 RPM units. The best, most durable generators and engines are the slower speed models. Their reserve capacity is greater, and breakdowns and repairs are fewer. Perhaps the only disability, other than a slightly higher cost, is the fact that the low RPM outfits are heavy.

When building a frame, keep this in mind. Balance the weight and spread the wheels enough so that capsizing is not a problem.

All of Jack's generators come with pre-wired panels. The only thing left to buy is a double pulley for the generator and two V belts. The engine comes with both a flat belt and V-belt pulley as standard equipment. Cost is nominal: less than fifty dollars. You can buy the pulley and belt locally or along with the engine. Since the precise speed at which the unit runs is important, I suggest get-

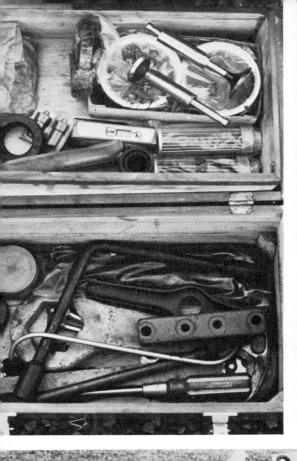
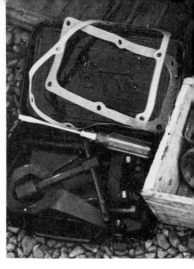
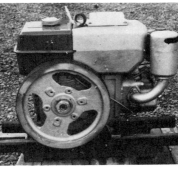
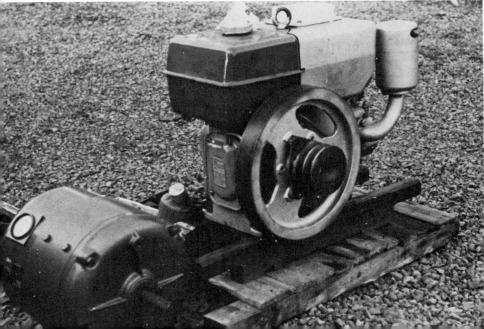

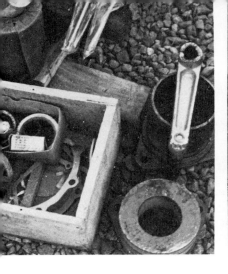
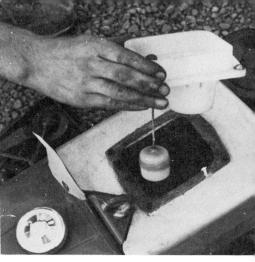

Photo at left shows 7-horsepower Chinese diesel engine, recommended as being the most fuel-efficient size for survivalists. Under full load, fuel consumption is less than one liter per hour. Each engine comes with a teakwood box filled with spare parts (*top left and center*), including filters, bearings, valve, injectors, sleeves, bolts, and numerous tools. Checking the water level (*top right*) is important, since water must be added to the engine every twelve hours or so to cool it. The manufacturer claims the engines will last for twenty-five years under normal usage. This 12-horsepower diesel (*bottom right*) is mounted on rails, and hooked up to an 8-kilowatt generator. Note the headlight; engine was originally made for a small Chinese tractor. Photo at bottom left illustrates a 7-horsepower engine ready to hook up to a 4-kilowatt generator. Unit will later be mounted on a metal skid, available from the Jack Bryant Company in Turner, Oregon.

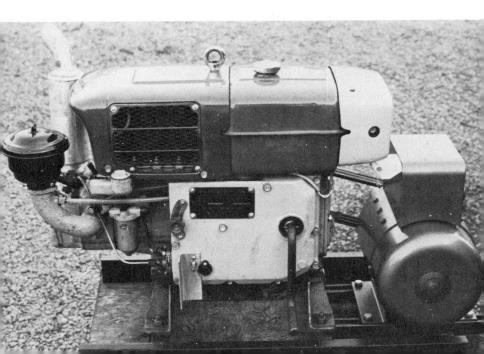

ting a pulley you know will be correct. I ordered mine with the engine and generator.

Problems

Like everything mechanical, breakdowns can occur. The generator should last for a minimum of twenty years. If it doesn't, virtually the only thing that could go wrong is worn-out bearings or brushes.

I suggest spending an extra twenty dollars on these spare parts. Hang them in a bag on the generator. It is cheap insurance against failure. All of the extra diesel parts and accessories one might need come with the engine as standard equipment. About the only extra parts I can think of for it might be a couple of fuel and air filters, costing less than ten dollars per set.

It has been my experience that some appliances suffer excess wear as a result of use on a home generation system. Unfortunately, freezers and water pumps are two of the most susceptible. They last about five years under these circumstances. Other than stocking up on freezer and pump motors, the only way I know of mitigating the problem is to start and stop the units as infrequently as possible.

I run my freezers continuously one hour twice a day while the generator is going, and that's it. When they come on, I watch that the first is running well before kicking in the second. Our pump goes till everything has water, and then shuts down for another twelve hours. There is but one start each time.

Hooking Up the Generator

Most power companies insist that home generators be hooked into the power system via a double throw box. The purpose of this very expensive piece of electrical equipment is to be sure no power is fed back out into the line while the generator is running.

My suggestion is that you rig a double-male plugged drop cord from the generator to a convenient 220 volt wall outlet. This can be a dryer, stove, or welder outlet. Wire in the correct plug to fit the generator panel on one end of a piece of number 8 wire and a plug to fit the appliance socket on the other.

As a precaution, pull the main fuses in your electrical box, as well as all of those controlling circuits that you plan not to use.

Putting the power through your own lines this way is much less expensive and troublesome than any other method I know of.

Other Uses for the Generator

I have my generator hooked up to my arc welder. At 4,000 watts, it doesn't have enough juice to run the welder full blast. However, it will handle 100 amps, which is good enough for most welding jobs.

A portable generator is an excellent survival tool for collecting fish from ponds and rivers. Two long leads can be strung from the 220 outlet to a hand-held pole. The ground wire must be placed well in the water. The leads on the poles become a probe in the water. Every fish swimming between the ground wire and the pole probe will immediately come rolling to the surface. If you are prudent, the larger fish can be taken without killing the smaller ones, leaving them to grow up.

19. A Simple A-Frame Cabin

Constructing good, serviceable survival buildings that are permanent in nature requires a lot of materials. One of the reasons we presently use dimension lumber and plywood for construction is because of the efficient use these materials make of our resources.

In a survival situation in the city, I believe there will be large quantities of conventional materials available to the scrounger. Construction under those circumstances will be pretty much a cut-and-paste situation, much the same as we know it today. Instead of going to the lumberyard, we will go down the street to some burned-out building for building materials.

Out in the country on private property and in the parks and national forests, it will be a no man's land. The raw materials will be there. It will become a matter of enforcing property rights more than anything else.

Assuming you have the raw materials plus the desire to build a home, it isn't terribly difficult to put up something pretty damn good. When I was younger, I used to build lean-to shelters or, as the Indians called them, *wickiups*. Perhaps it's that early experience that is still influencing me today, because I am very partial to A-frame cabin construction in the woods.

There are, of course, many other types of cabins that can be built out of logs, using rough construction techniques, and rudimentary tools. Some are very good and perhaps deserve a mention in this book. Yet there are some logical reasons for sticking with one design.

A-Frame Advantages

The principal advantage when constructing an A-frame is that the structure is ideally suited to the use of rough, raw materials with irregular dimensions. It is also a simple house to build, and is

246

ready to live in as soon as the walls are raised. The design is such that the builder can display a generous amount of ineptitude and still come out with a usable building. Also, not to be forgotten, an A-frame is heat efficient, an important attribute.

Materials List for 18' x 30' A-frame

Here's what you'll need to make my A-frame:

3   24-inch diameter foundation posts 11 feet long. (Assumes foundation will have a center support.)

2   24-inch diameter side foundation posts 8½ feet long. (Assumes sides will be split run.)

20   Or so medium rocks to support posts.

3   Large rocks for back supports.

2   18-inch x 10-foot front floor support beams.

6   20-inch x 15-foot floor joist beams.

45   12-inch diameter logs 9 feet long, split in half, used for floor of deck.

22   9-inch base diameter tapering logs 17 feet long, 2 each used for making A's.

11   8-inch diameter split logs for lower crosspieces on A's, about 10 feet long.

11   8-inch diameter split logs for top A crosspieces. These can be scrap about 4 feet long.

1,000   Running feet of 3-inch poles for roof slats.

2,000   Sq. ft. of shingles, assuming a half overlap.

6   12-inch logs 12 feet long, split in half for the loft floor.

900   Running feet of 4-inch poles used to cover the ends of the house.

800   Sq. ft. of shingles to cover ends.

Materials for ladders, counter, etc.:

100   Lbs. 12-penny nails.

50   Lbs. 20-penny nails.

25   Lbs. #16 black wire.

Shovel, chain saw, heavy hammer, bubble level,
maul, ax, wedges, square, heavy string, hand saw,
and pliers.

Site Selection

Let's assume you have the necessary tools and materials, plus a
whole forest full of trees. Locate a gently sloping piece of ground
that is level side to side. The site should slope away about 5 feet
from the back of the cabin to the front; i.e., if the cabin is 30 feet
long, ideally the rear floor will rest level on the ground while the
front is about 5 feet off the ground when level.

You can make this determination using a bubble level and a
piece of string stretched taut between a peg in the ground and a
pole.

Floor and Foundation

Eighteen feet is about an ideal width for a small A-frame cabin.
There are many other good reasons this is true, but for the present,
just the fact that it will only take 9-foot lengths of floor material to
span beam to center beam is important. Larger logs are desperately
hard to split evenly.

Bury to a depth of 6 feet two heavy 11-foot post logs in the
ground on the downhill side of the house. Using your string as a
level, cut these foundation posts off evenly. These posts must be
very substantial. Space them out so that they are about 8 inches
farther apart than the intended width of the house on each side.
Put in a center foundation post if needed.

Place a very heavy solid floor support log on the posts. Since the
A-frame is 18 feet wide, you will not be able to lift this log. Using
a peavey, roll it uphill and then back down on two logs set at an
incline on the posts. Sometimes it isn't practical to run a single
floor support log across 18 feet. If you used three foundation posts,
you will need two 9-foot floor support logs.

Length of the house must already have been determined when
the land was initially surveyed. To a great extent, the availability of
materials will dictate this. If you have the logs and the energy,
make the house 30 feet deep as indicated. If not, make it 20. I like to
split the run and put in a center foundation post on each side. That

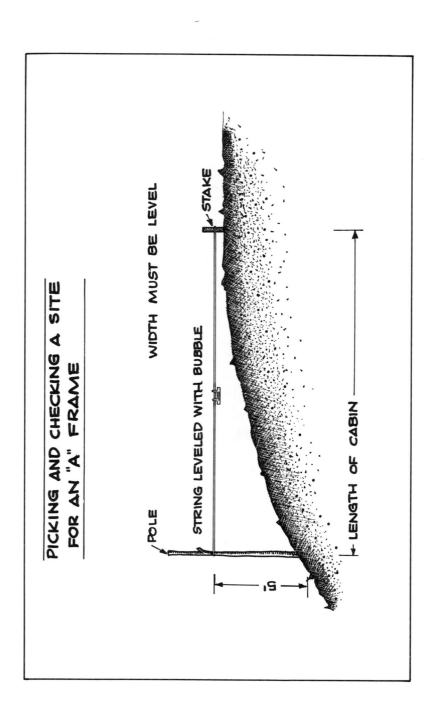

PICKING AND CHECKING A SITE FOR AN "A" FRAME

WIDTH MUST BE LEVEL

STAKE

STRING LEVELED WITH BUBBLE

POLE

5'

LENGTH OF CABIN

way I can use two 10-foot or two 15-foot side floor beams instead of one long one.

Any floor (or deck) support beams used must be very heavy and very sound. Don't skimp here. Use the biggest beams you have and can roll up on the support posts. Be sure the tops of the supports are level with the world and with each other. This isn't hard if you use logs that are close in diameter, and plan ahead a bit. Look at the drawing for ideas.

Cabin Floor

I use wedges and a maul to split cedar for the floor. If that isn't available, use birch if you can get it, hackberry if you can find long enough pieces, or whatever is available in your area. In the West where I live now, the best by far is tamarack.

It is very difficult to get the logs to split evenly and lie straight with one another on the decks. You may waste a lot of wood and time putting the deck in correctly. Don't leave gaping holes unless you have plywood or some kind of boards to finish the floor with. Holes in the floor let the cold in. A good, thick layer of tamarack is an excellent insulator.

I use logs that are about 12 inches in diameter for my floor if possible. Bigger or smaller are fine if you can acquire the knack of splitting them to yield a deck member that is about the same as the others.

A-Support Beams

Once the deck is completed, you are ready to start building the A supports. I usually do the rest of the necessary carpentry on the deck itself. It's a nice flat place to build the A supports, which can be stacked on the ground alongside as they are built.

If the building is to be made completely of rough materials, I space the A supports 3 feet apart, using eleven A's on a 30-foot run. It's a matter of personal preference, but I like the finished building to have roof walls 1 foot shorter than the width of the base. In the case of an 18-foot deck, the A supports would then be 17 feet long. This is a good length in many woods. Nice straight ash or pine trees can be found that are long enough.

Use A support poles that are trimmed to about 9 inches at the base tapering to no less than 5 inches at the top end.

SIDE VIEW OF DECK
SUPPORTS AND DECK

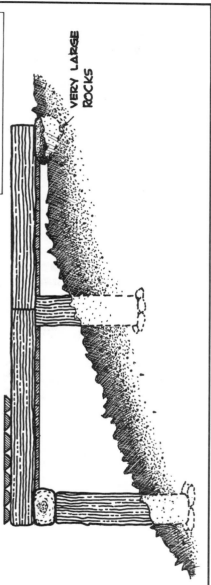

POST SUPPORTS
(FRONT VIEW)

TRIM CROSSPIECE SO IT LIES LEVEL

FRONT POSTS
MUST BE
VERY
HEAVY

SET POSTS
ABOUT
8"
WIDER
THAN
HOUSE

POSTS CUT OFF LEVEL
(ABOUT FIVE FEET)

CENTER POST OPTIONAL ON
WIDTHS LESS THAN 18'

LARGE ROCKS KEEP POSTS FROM SINKING

9'

VERY LARGE
ROCKS

DECK FLOOR MADE OF SPLIT POLES

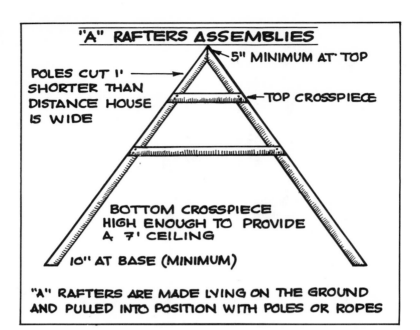

"A" RAFTERS ASSEMBLIES

5" MINIMUM AT TOP

POLES CUT 1'
SHORTER THAN
DISTANCE HOUSE
IS WIDE

TOP CROSSPIECE

BOTTOM CROSSPIECE
HIGH ENOUGH TO PROVIDE
A 7' CEILING

10" AT BASE (MINIMUM)

"A" RAFTERS ARE MADE LYING ON THE GROUND
AND PULLED INTO POSITION WITH POLES OR ROPES

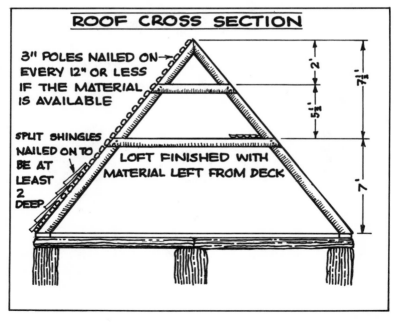

ROOF CROSS SECTION

3" POLES NAILED ON
EVERY 12" OR LESS
IF THE MATERIAL
IS AVAILABLE

2'

7½'

5½'

SPLIT SHINGLES
NAILED ON TO
BE AT
LEAST
2"
DEEP.

LOFT FINISHED WITH
MATERIAL LEFT FROM DECK

7'

The roof peak under these circumstances will be 14½ feet from the surface of the deck. This is a really good practical working distance. It provides room for a loft inside, but is not so high that it is impossible to work on the building without sky hooks.

Lay out the A's on the deck. Carefully cut the poles and trim the ends. Then lay in 8-inch diameter crosspieces and nail and/or wire securely. The crosspiece will be about 10 feet long. Level them on a mark 8 feet 3 inches up on the main A beams. This will provide a ceiling for the first floor 7 feet high.

The crosspieces can be of irregular material. They are leveled from the top so other than the fact that you will have to look at irregular floor supports, it doesn't make much difference. I use the scrap left from the deck.

Nail the 4-feet-long top crosspieces 2 feet 3 inches down from the top of the A's. This allows enough room for a 5-foot 6-inch ceiling in the sleeping loft. All the sleeping is done in the loft of an A-frame because that's where the heat is. Lofts can also be used for storage and as a place to dry things. Their only problem is they tend to be very dark.

Put the A's up on 3-foot centers (3 feet apart). If some poles are wider than others, it won't matter. Nail the A's securely on the side floor joists and fasten to 3-inch roof poles running along the side on top.

All of the roof poles should be nailed on after the A's are erected. I like to use maple or oak roof poles, or lodgepole pine in the West works well. Split cedar also works. Pieces 3 inches by 9 feet long are ideal if you can get them.

Use lots of this material. A run every 12 inches is none too much if you can do it.

Making Cedar Shingles

Personally I like thick-split cedar shingles for the roof; if not cedar, then tamarack or hackberry. Even old boards will work for many, many years. The roof is so steep that the overlapped boards will keep the cabin dry, even if there are large holes showing. Use thick shingles, greatly overlapped, if you can do it. This is important because of the good insulating qualities of a heavier roof.

I have heard of grass or pine bough roofs on A-frames, but think the idea may be impractical. This sort of roofing would deteriorate very quickly.

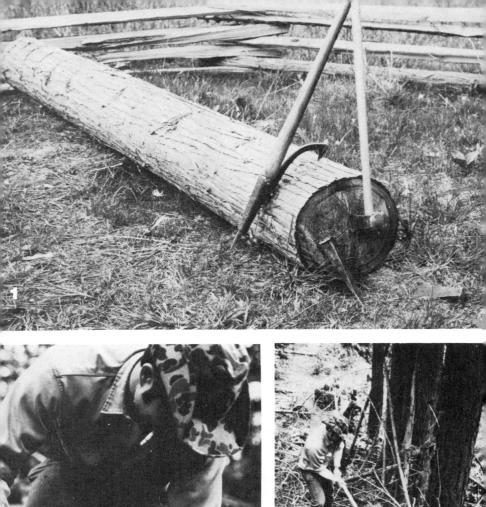

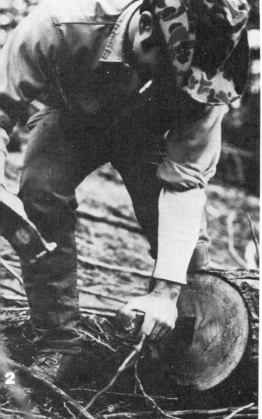

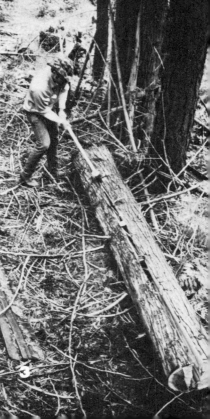

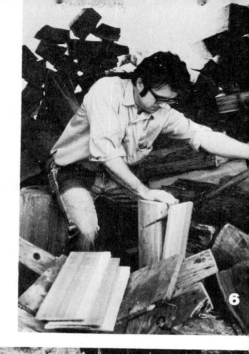

Photo sequence demonstrates how to make split poles for deck or cedar shingles. (*1*) The materials needed for shingle-making: wedges, a peavey, a maul-ax, and cedar log. (*2*) Log is split in half starting from end, (*3*) Using wedges and maul-ax, log is split progressively up its entire length. (*4 & 5*) To complete splitting, peavey is used to pry the two log-halves apart. Each half is cut into 3-foot blocks, and bark removed (*not shown*). Photo *6* illustrates shakes being cut from blocks. This cutting is done with the grain, using a heavy, long-bladed knife and wedges, or a special shake knife as shown.

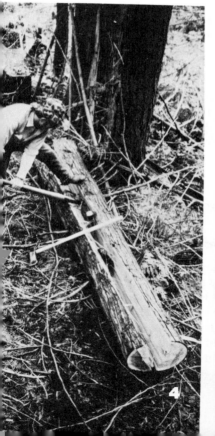

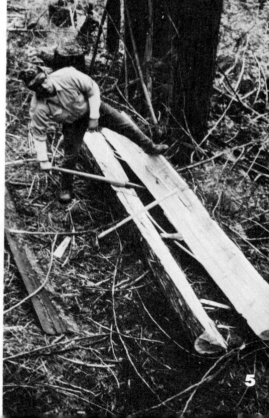

Split cedar shingles about 10 inches wide, 3 feet long, and 2 inches thick are ideal. Even if the shingles are not tapered, they work the best of anything. See the cedar-shingle-making photo series for details of this process.

Finishing

Finish the loft floor the same way you did the main floor, using the same material, if possible. Try to make a thinner, lighter floor than the main deck. Often the loft deck is only put in over two-thirds of the main living area below.

The ends of the house should be set in 3 feet. As a result, the inside floor space will be cut down from a 30-foot length to 24 feet. However, the 3-foot overhangs are extremely useful. They are ideal places to store firewood, hang deer, keep tools, leave one's boots, tie the dog, or smoke and dry food.

Close the two cabin ends with 4-inch poles nailed side by side vertically. Leave a space 2½ feet wide by 6½ feet high on both ends for doors. Doors can be made out of 6-inch pole frames wet deer skin tacked to the frame. The drying skin gets tight as a drum and holds the frame together.

Windows on an A-frame are a problem. If you can, salvage some from an old barn or home and build them into the ends. A-frames are dark anyway. Without windows they are really dreary.

I like to chink the end logs with mud and then shingle over the whole thing. This makes a very nice warm wall, if the shingles are available.

A ladder should be provided up to the deck in front. The entire lower living area can be lined with firewood or other storage items to provide more insulation.

Heating Sources

The best heat comes, in my opinion, from a stove. If you are a stonemason, or bricklayer, you could put in a fireplace. However, if you do, put the fireplace inside the house as a freestanding unit. Do not build it on an end wall or into a side wall.

Fireplaces are notoriously inefficient. If one is put against an outside wall, it will draw in cold from the outside rather than heat the place. A freestanding unit will heat the rock of the chimney, providing warmth after the fire goes out.

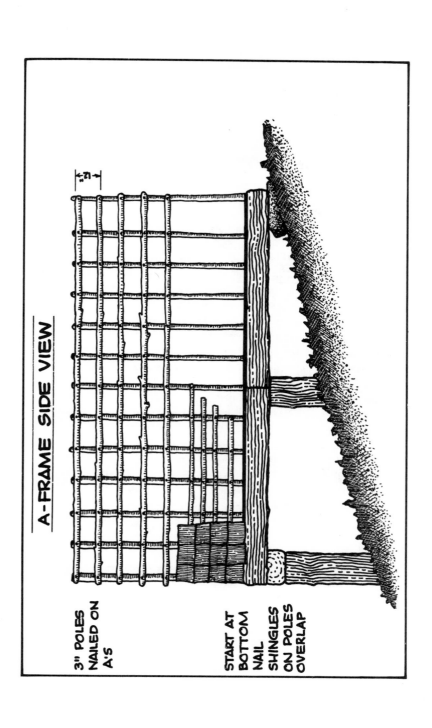

A-FRAME SIDE VIEW

3" POLES
NAILED ON
A'S

START AT
BOTTOM
NAIL
SHINGLES
ON POLES
OVERLAP

"A" FRAME FRONT VIEW

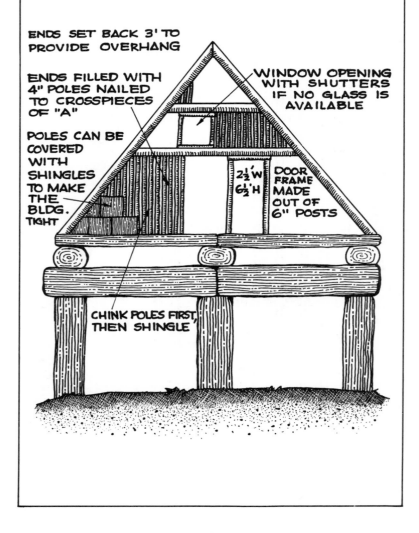

ENDS SET BACK 3' TO PROVIDE OVERHANG

ENDS FILLED WITH 4" POLES NAILED TO CROSSPIECES OF "A"

POLES CAN BE COVERED WITH SHINGLES TO MAKE THE BLDG. TIGHT

WINDOW OPENING WITH SHUTTERS IF NO GLASS IS AVAILABLE

2½' W
6½' H

DOOR FRAME MADE OUT OF 6" POSTS

CHINK POLES FIRST THEN SHINGLE

Stoves don't look as nice in an A-frame as fireplaces, but they are far more efficient and practical. A small wood cook stove will keep an A-frame like this one nice and warm on three cords of wood a year. If a cast iron stove is not available, make a stove out of a steel 55-gallon drum, using coffee cans for stovepipe. This job requires a welder or a very patient man with a cold chisel and hammer.

Put plumbing in the cabin to suit yourself. A-frames of this type that I have built have had outhouses. The facility was located out the back door to the left. Not all that inconvenient, even in the dead of winter.

Water

You must, under any circumstances, plan ahead for water. Before cutting down the first tree, figure out where water is going to come from.

My favorite technique is to develop a spring. Doing this requires using pipe of some kind or another. If you are unable to obtain pipe, it isn't practical to have running water in the house.

The spring being developed must be located uphill from the A-frame. In actual practice, it needn't be all that close. One spring we tapped was fifteen hundred feet from the house, which in case you missed it, was over a quarter of a mile away.

Dig down into the spring at least 4 feet, setting boards up as a dam or barrier. At the bottom, drill a hole in the board the size of your pipe and run it downhill to the cabin. At the cabin you can rig a shutoff, or run the water into a barrel.

Electrical Wiring

If you plan for electricity, put the generator under the front deck, or in its own shelter off to the side. Generators are noisy, smelly, and unsociable, but must be kept out of the weather.

Usually A-frames are wired from one side, up the top, over and down the other side, rather than room by room as in conventional houses. This leads to some odd circuits, such as a crawl space light, first floor front outlet, upstairs outlet, upstairs light, for instance, all on one circuit. Not doing it this way will result in the use of an inordinate amount of wire, even in a little survival cabin.

Time Requirements

Here is how I would break down the time and chores needed to complete my 18-by-30-foot A-frame cabin. The list of tasks assumes one has a reasonable location with good timber near at hand. In addition, I am assuming there are two motivated, healthy people available to do the work who have access to a chain saw. This list is the approximate length of time it took my wife and me to build an A-frame under the conditions described. We were in good physical shape at the time.

Develop spring and run 1-inch plastic pipe for 1,000 feet, 18 inches underground, to the cabin site	2 days
Set foundation poles and put floor supports and joists in place	2 days
Split logs for deck and set in place	4 days
Gather materials and construct 11 A's for the roof and walls	3 days
Set up A's	1 day
Nail A's together with roof poles	3 days
Split out cedar or tamarack shingles and put on roof	13 days
Put in end walls, using old barn doors and windows. Ends were shingles with rejects from roof.	8 days
Build in loft	2 days
Ladders, railings, and other miscellany	4 days
Stove and stovepipe	3 days
Electrical wiring (optional)	3 days

In total, plan on about two months' labor before you can move in and stay warm and dry. After that, it will take at least a year to build a root cellar, clear and plow a garden, stack wood, construct an outhouse, make some furniture, set some trap lines, get the water to where it is a bit handier, and generally make the place livable.

All of this requires a whole bunch of extremely hard work. It's sobering for me to look back and realize how hard our forefathers really did work just to stay alive. Very few people in this country are going to be able to do it again. If you are some of the people who can, I wish you well. I believe life will, in the truest sort of way, be very rewarding for you.

20. Real Survivors

People who make rash predictions, whether economic, social, political, or religious, are fools. The world is full of false messiahs who, having led their followers up the hill in triumph, are forced to come down again the next morning.

It was with trepidation that I accepted an invitation to meet with some European retirees who were visiting this country for the first time. Perhaps two weeks remained before the completion of this book. I was extremely busy, and was not too interested in playing tour-guide for some strange tourists.

At the meeting, I was introduced to folks like old Ingle. From northern Germany and almost eighty-five, he was a survivor of both world wars. Irmgard, his wife, is not yet seventy, but she remembers Rumania when she was young. "There wasn't a blade of grass near our home," she says. "The only people who made it either had lots of food in storage or something very valuable to trade. We ate the leaves off the trees. There wasn't even enough grass to feed our rabbits. By the second year we ate them all, rather than let them starve," she continued.

Barta, an old friend of my father's, remembered without fondness a barrel of cod liver oil his family had stored. For months on end they lived on little else.

The group of old survivors talked about the wormy potatoes, the scarcity of meat, and the sawdust in the bread. The picture they painted was incredibly grim.

The visitors never suspected that I was finishing a book on surviving life as they described it. To be involved in that conversation was a vindication. It reconfirmed my belief that my advice was good. People could indeed live with it.

"You have debased your currency, destroyed your productive capacity, and enslaved the producers," Barta said. "It's no good. You will pay the price. You Americans are like the Soviets. Sitting on a wealth of energy and raw materials that politically might as well be on the moon. The politicians will sell you out and starve you," he quietly intoned, "but perhaps some will live if they have the will."

The next day my friends continued on their tour. "The old folks didn't make it," they reminded me before leaving. "It was just too rough. For you Americans, it's going to be hell."

I'm not a young man. But perhaps you can do it, if you are tough. At least you can't say you weren't taught how.

Publisher's note: Ragnar Benson welcomes correspondence from his readers. If you have an old-time technique you'd like to share, or any questions or suggestions, drop a line to Ragnar Benson, c/o Paladin Press Editorial Dept., P.O. Box 1307, Boulder, Colorado 80306. Your cards and letters will be greatly appreciated.